# 100+ Keto Chaffle Recipes

# Table of Contents

# Disclaimer

# Introduction

Eating healthy is critical to our very existence. A hearty meal will energize you through the toughest of days. Many people skip meals like breakfast because they're either too busy or trying to lose weight. However, this is definitely not the way to go. This book will give you a much healthier alternative and sustainable solution.

So let's talk about waffles. Do you love waffles? Are they your favorite breakfast meal? Well, you're not alone. However, traditional waffles are generally cut from the diet when you want to lose weight. They're high in carbs and not a good option if you've put on those extra pounds. However, we have a solution for you, and they're called keto chaffles. These are a much better alternative compared to how you usually make your waffles. As you read on, you'll learn what going keto means and what keto chaffles are.

## About Keto Chaffles

First, let's understand what the term keto means. Keto is short for ketogenic, and it's a diet where you eat more fats. This may seem contradictory to your purpose if you're trying to lose weight, but it really does work. Fats are not as bad as they're made out to be. Instead of cutting out all the fatty foods that you usually like to eat, you have to cut down on carbohydrates drastically. The modern diet is loaded with carbohydrates, and this is one of the main reasons for the rise in weight issues. The incidence of obesity and diseases like diabetes type 2 is much more prevalent in our generation than in that of our ancestors. This is because they ate a healthier diet with wholesome natural foods. The modern diet is filled with processed foods that have preservatives and many hidden ingredients that are harmful to health. Refined sugar is amongst the worst things that we eat, as it has no nutritional value and can cause immense harm to health. People have been becoming much more conscious of their dietary choices lately. It is quite evident that the current food choices that most people make have done nothing beneficial for their health. This is why everyone is looking for a healthy alternative that will help them lose weight as well. Unfortunately, people get taken in by the false promises of many fad diets. Such diets will ask them to skip meals, eat only liquids, give up all fatty foods, etc. None of these are healthy and sustainable options. They harm the body in many ways. You may lose a little weight, but then you'll gain it again. However, we have a solution for you.

The ketogenic diet is effective and healthy for everyone. This book will help you get started with recipes for keto-friendly breakfast waffles that we call chaffles. Chaffles are made with eggs and cheese. These are healthy fats that are keto-friendly.

You won't be using the normal carbohydrate-laden ingredients that are usually used for making waffles. This will allow you to enjoy waffles without worrying about gaining weight. It's incredible how you can enjoy so many of your favorite foods when you go keto, but you still get the benefits of eating healthy. When you try out the keto chaffle recipes in this book, you'll probably tempt a lot of people around you to go keto as well.

Chaffles are not just for breakfast; you can enjoy them for other meals as well. So now you can enjoy some toasty chaffles whenever you want and not worry about missing out on your favorite food. Keto alternatives for any recipe can be really great for your health.

So without any further ado, let us get started.

# Few Tips For Making Perfect Chaffles

- Read the manufacturer's instructions carefully from the instructions manual. Every manufacture is different so the instructions may vary.
- Adding a tablespoon of almond flour (per egg) to the basic recipe will help make better, crispier chaffles.
- Heat the waffle maker before pouring the batter in the waffle maker. If it is not preheated, the ingredients may get stuck to it. It is preferable to heat the waffle iron between 2 chaffles as well.
- Brush some oil in the waffle maker after the waffle maker is heated. You can also spray with cooking spray. This is common for all the recipes unless specified otherwise and will not be mentioned in every recipe.
- Whisk eggs and cheese well. Eggs should be at room temperature. Other ingredients should also be at room temperature unless specified otherwise.
- Do not pour more than 2 to 4 tablespoons of the batter in a mini waffle maker. It will spill out and make a mess. You can place the waffle maker on a silicone or silpat mat so that any spills can be collected on it.
- Spread the batter evenly in the waffle maker.

- Scatter a little cheese, preferably mozzarella cheese (apart from what is mentioned in the recipe) on the waffle maker initially. The cheese should cover the bottom of the waffle maker. Next pour the egg mixture. Sprinkle some more cheese over the egg mixture.
- Remember to set the timer if your waffle maker does not have an automatic timer.
- Place cooked chaffles in an air fryer to keep warm if necessary.
- To make crispy chaffles, use only whites of the eggs. When you take out the chaffles from the waffle maker, set aside for a few minutes. It will crisp up. Also it becomes crisp if you cook for a longer time.
- For extra crisp chaffles, place them in the toaster or oven. You can also add a little butter into a skillet and heat the chaffles until it becomes extra crisp.
- Be patient while making the chaffles. If it is not done in the set time, cook for some more time until it is crisp.
- Shallow waffle iron will give crisper waffles.
- You can pour the eggs in a squeeze bottle to pour into the waffle maker if desired.
- Do not keep opening the waffle maker every few minutes to check. It will delay the cooking of the chaffle. In fact do not open until the set time.

- If you do not like a cheesy taste, use mozzarella cheese. You can also use goat's cheese or halloumi cheese.
- You can use cream cheese instead of mozzarella cheese for sweet chaffles.
- You can make extra chaffles and store in an airtight container in the refrigerator. It can last for 5 to 6 days. You can reheat in a toaster or oven or a pan with a little butter.
- You can try making variations with ingredients of your choice.

# Few Tips On Cleaning The Waffle Maker

- For non-removable plates: Firstly unplug the waffle maker. Let it cool until slightly warm or cool completely but it cleans better when the waffle maker is warm.
- Remove any bits and pieces of chaffle if any.
- First wipe with a paper towel to remove any extra oil. Fold the paper towel because it will more absorb oil.
- Moisten a piece of cotton cloth or a paper towel and clean the waffle make while the waffle maker is still slightly warm. It becomes easier to clean up. Wipe inside as well as outside. If the waffle maker is completely cooled, dip a kitchen cloth in hot water and squeeze a little to drain off excess water and clean the waffle maker. Let the moisture remain it in for 4 – 5 minutes.
- Clean the grooves of the waffle maker with a spatula. Use a toothbrush with soft bristles for stubborn, stuck particles. If it still does not come off, brush some oil on the food particles. Wipe off after about 15 minutes with a piece of cloth dipped in warm soap solution. Rinse the cloth and wipe again.
- Wipe the outside for the waffle maker as well.
- Do not immerse the waffle iron in water.

- For removable plates: Immerse the plates in a bowl of water. Let it soak for a few minutes. Clean with a sponge or toothbrush with soft bristles. Wipe the outside of the waffle maker.
- Wipe with a dry cloth. Let it dry for a while on your countertop. Place the plates back in the waffle maker.

# Chapter 1: Keto Chaffle Recipes

## Basic Keto Chaffle #1

Makes: 4 chaffles

**Ingredients:**

- 1 cup finely shredded mozzarella cheese
- 2 large eggs

To serve:

- Melted butter
- Sugar-free syrup

**Directions:**

1. Preheat the mini waffle maker.
2. Beat eggs with a fork. Stir in the mozzarella.
3. Spoon ¼ of the batter into the waffle maker. Set the timer for 2 to 3 minutes. Close the waffle maker.
4. Take out the chaffle and set aside on a plate. Let it sit for a couple of minutes.
5. Repeat steps 3 – 4 and make the remaining chaffles.

6. Brush with some melted butter. Drizzle some sugar-free syrup on top and serve.

## Basic Keto Chaffle #2

Makes: 4 chaffles

**Ingredients:**

- 1 cup finely shredded cheddar cheese
- 2 large eggs
- 4 tablespoons almond flour

To serve:

- Melted butter
- Sugar-free syrup

**Directions:**

1. Preheat the mini waffle maker.
2. Beat eggs with a fork. Stir in cheddar cheese and almond flour.
3. Spoon ¼ of the batter into the waffle maker. Set the timer for 3- 4 minutes. Close the waffle maker.

4. Take out the chaffle and set aside on a plate. Let it sit for a couple of minutes.
5. Repeat steps 3 – 4 and make the remaining chaffles.
6. Brush with some melted butter. Drizzle some sugar-free syrup on top and serve.

# Basic Keto Chaffle #3

Makes: 4 chaffles

## Ingredients:

- 1 cup finely shredded mozzarella cheese
- 2 eggs
- 4 tablespoons almond flour
- ½ teaspoon baking powder
- 1 teaspoon psyllium husk powder

To serve:

- Melted butter
- Sugar-free syrup

## Directions:

1. Preheat the mini waffle maker.
2. Beat eggs with a fork.
3. Add almond flour, baking powder and psyllium husk powder into a bowl and stir until well combined. Add into the bowl of eggs. Whisk well.
4. Stir in mozzarella cheese.
7. Spoon ¼ of the batter into the waffle maker. Set the timer for about 6 - 8 minutes. Close the waffle maker.

5. Check after about 5 minutes. Cook until crisp.
6. Take out the chaffle and set aside on a plate. Let it sit for a couple of minutes.
7. Repeat steps 5 – 6 and make the remaining chaffles.
8. Brush with some melted butter. Drizzle some sugar-free syrup on top and serve.

## Vegan Keto Chaffle

Makes: 4 chaffles

### Ingredients:

- 2 tablespoons flaxseed meal
- ½ cup shredded low carb vegan cheese
- 2 tablespoons low carb vegan cream cheese, softened
- 5 tablespoons water
- 4 tablespoons coconut flour
- A pinch salt

### Directions:

1. Plug in the waffle maker and let it preheat.
2. Add flaxseed meal and water into a bowl and whisk well. Set aside for 10 – 15 minutes. This is the flax egg.
3. Add vegan cheese, vegan cream cheese, coconut flour and water into the bowl of flax eggs and whisk well.

4. Spoon ¼ of the batter into the waffle maker. Set the timer for about 5 minutes. Close the waffle maker.
5. Check after about 4 – 5 minutes. Cook until crisp if desired.
6. Take out the chaffle and set aside on a plate. Let it sit for a couple of minutes.
7. Repeat steps 4 – 6 and make the remaining chaffles.

# Cinnamon Chaffle

Makes: 4 Chaffles

## Ingredients:

- 2 cups finely shredded mozzarella cheese
- 2 eggs
- 2 tablespoons almond flour
- 2 teaspoons vanilla extract
- 2 teaspoons baking powder
- ½ teaspoon ground cinnamon

To serve:

- Melted butter
- Sugar-free syrup

## Directions:

1. Preheat the mini waffle maker.
2. Beat eggs with a fork. Add vanilla and whisk well.
3. Add almond flour, baking powder and cinnamon into a bowl and stir until well combined. Add into the bowl of eggs. Stir until well combined.
4. Stir in mozzarella cheese.

8. Spoon ¼ of the batter into the waffle maker. Set the timer for about 5 – 6 minutes. Close the waffle maker.

5. Check after about 5 minutes. Cook until crisp.

6. Take out the chaffle when cooked and set aside on a plate. Let it sit for a couple of minutes.

7. Repeat steps 5 – 6 and make the remaining chaffles.

8. Brush with some melted butter. Drizzle some sugar-free syrup on top and serve.

# Cream Cheese Chaffle

Makes: 3 chaffles

## Ingredients:

- 1 egg
- 1 tablespoon almond flour
- ½ teaspoon baking powder
- ½ cup shredded mozzarella cheese
- 1 tablespoon cream cheese, softened
- 1 ½ tablespoons water (optional)

## Directions:

1. Add egg into a bowl and beat with a fork.
2. Add almond flour, baking powder, mozzarella cheese, cream cheese and water and whisk well.
3. Spoon ½ of the batter into the waffle maker. Set the timer for 3- 4 minutes. Close the waffle maker.
4. Take out the chaffle and set aside on a plate. Let it sit for a couple of minutes.
5. Repeat steps 3 – 4 and make the remaining chaffles.
6. Brush some melted butter on top and serve.

# Cinnamon Sugar (Churro) Chaffle

Makes: 4 – 5 Chaffles

## Ingredients:

- 1 ½ cups finely shredded mozzarella cheese
- 1 tablespoon butter, melted
- 4 tablespoons erythritol
- 2 large eggs
- 4 tablespoons blanched almond flour
- 1 teaspoon vanilla extract
- ½ teaspoon baking powder (optional)
- 1 teaspoon psyllium husk powder (optional)
- 1 teaspoon ground cinnamon

To serve:

- Melted butter
- Ground cinnamon
- Erythritol

## Directions:

1. Preheat the mini waffle maker.
2. Beat eggs with a fork. Add vanilla and whisk well.

3. Add almond flour, psyllium husk, baking powder, erythritol and cinnamon into a bowl and stir until well combined. Add into the bowl of eggs. Whisk well.

4. Stir in mozzarella cheese.

5. Spoon about ¼ of the batter into the waffle maker. Set the timer for about 10 minutes. Close the waffle maker.

6. Check after about 5 minutes. Cook until crisp.

7. Take out the chaffle and set aside on a plate. Let it sit for a couple of minutes.

8. Repeat steps 5 – 6 and make the remaining chaffles.

9. Brush with some melted butter. Mix together erythritol, and cinnamon in a bowl. Sprinkle on top of the chaffles and serve and serve.

# Pumpkin Chaffle

Makes: 4 – 5

## Ingredients:

- 1 cup finely shredded mozzarella cheese
- 1 ounce cream cheese
- ½ tablespoon pumpkin pie spice
- 5 tablespoons erythritol
- 2 large eggs
- 4 tablespoons pumpkin puree
- 1 teaspoon vanilla extract (optional)
- ½ teaspoon baking powder (optional)
- 6 teaspoons coconut flour

## Directions:

1. Preheat the mini waffle maker.
2. Beat eggs with a fork. Add vanilla, pumpkin puree and cream cheese and whisk well.
3. Add coconut flour, baking powder, erythritol and pumpkin pie spice into a bowl and stir until well combined. Add into the bowl of egg mixture. Mix until well combined.
4. Stir in mozzarella cheese.

5. Spoon about 4 – 5 tablespoons of the batter into the waffle maker. Set the timer for about 6 – 8 minutes. Close the waffle maker.

6. Check after about 5 minutes. Cook until crisp.

7. Take out the chaffle and set aside on a plate. Let it sit for a couple of minutes.

8. Repeat steps 5 – 6 and make the remaining chaffles.

9. Brush with some melted butter and serve.

# Chocolate Chaffle

Makes: 2

## Ingredients:

- 1 large egg
- ¼ teaspoon + 1/8 teaspoon baking powder
- 2 tablespoons very fine blanched almond flour
- ½ cup shredded cheese
- 1 tablespoon cacao powder or unsweetened cocoa powder
- 1 tablespoon swerve or erythritol
- ¼ teaspoon vanilla extract
- 1 tablespoon sugar-free chocolate chips

## Directions:

1. Preheat the mini waffle maker.
2. Beat egg with a fork. Add vanilla, almond flour, baking powder, erythritol and cocoa into a bowl and stir until well combined.
3. Stir in mozzarella cheese and chocolate chips.
4. Spoon ½ the batter into the waffle maker. Set the timer for about 6 – 8 minutes. Close the waffle maker.
5. Flip sides after about 5 minutes. Cook until crisp.

6.  Take out the chaffle and set aside on a plate. Let it sit for a couple of minutes.
7.  Repeat steps 4 – 6 and make the remaining chaffles.

# Caramel Chaffle

Makes: 4 chaffles

## Ingredients:

### For chaffle:

- 2/3 cup finely shredded mozzarella cheese
- 2 eggs
- 4 tablespoons almond flour
- 2 tablespoons swerve confectioners
- 1 teaspoon vanilla extract

### For caramel sauce:

- 6 tablespoons unsalted butter
- 2/3 cup heavy whipping cream
- 4 tablespoons swerve brown substitute
- 1 teaspoon vanilla extract

## Directions:

1. To make caramel: Place a skillet over medium heat. Add butter and swerve and stir occasionally until the mixture starts caramelizing.
2. Whisk in the cream and cook until thick. Turn off the heat and stir in vanilla.

3. Preheat the mini waffle maker.

4. Beat eggs with a fork.

5. Add almond flour and swerve into a bowl and stir until well combined. Add into the bowl of eggs. Whisk well.

6. Stir in mozzarella cheese.

7. Spoon ¼ of the batter into the waffle maker. Set the timer for about 6 - 8 minutes. Close the waffle maker.

8. Check after about 5 minutes. Cook until crisp if desired.

9. Take out the chaffle and set aside on a plate. Let it sit for a couple of minutes.

10. Repeat steps 7 – 9 and make the remaining chaffles.

11. Brush with some melted butter. Drizzle some caramel sauce on top and serve

Almond Butter Chaffles

Makes: 2

## Ingredients:

- 1 large egg
- ¼ teaspoon + 1/8 teaspoon baking powder
- 2 tablespoons very fine blanched almond flour
- ½ cup shredded cheese
- 2 tablespoons almond butter
- 1 tablespoon swerve or erythritol
- ¼ teaspoon vanilla extract

## Directions:

1. Add almond butter into a microwave safe bowl. Microwave on high for 20 seconds or until softened.
2. Preheat the mini waffle maker.
3. Beat egg with a fork. Add almond butter and whisk well. Add vanilla, almond flour, baking powder and erythritol into a bowl and stir until well combined.
4. Stir in mozzarella cheese.
5. Spoon ½ the batter into the waffle maker. Set the timer for about 6 – 8 minutes. Close the waffle maker.
6. Flip sides after about 5 minutes. Cook until crisp.

7. Take out the chaffle and set aside on a plate. Let it sit for a couple of minutes.
8. Repeat steps 5 – 7 and make the remaining chaffle.

# Blueberry Chaffle

Makes: 2 – 3

## Ingredients:

- ½ cup finely shredded mozzarella cheese
- 1 egg
- 1 tablespoon almond flour
- 1 teaspoon swerve sweetener
- ½ teaspoon baking powder
- ½ teaspoon ground cinnamon
- 1 ½ tablespoons blueberries

To serve:

- Melted butter
- Sugar-free syrup

## Directions:

1. Preheat the mini waffle maker.
2. Beat egg with a fork. Add vanilla and whisk well.
3. Add almond flour, baking powder, swerve and cinnamon into a bowl and stir until well combined. Add into the bowl of eggs. Mix well.
4. Stir in mozzarella cheese and blueberries.

5. Spoon 4 – 5 tablespoons of the batter into the waffle maker. Set the timer for about 6 – 7 minutes. Close the waffle maker.
6. Check after about 5 minutes. Cook until crisp.
7. Take out the chaffle and set aside on a plate. Let it sit for a couple of minutes.
8. Repeat steps 5 – 6 and make the remaining chaffles.
9. Brush with some melted butter. Drizzle some sugar-free syrup on top and serve.

# Cinnamon Roll Keto Chaffle

Makes: 6

**Ingredients:**

<u>For cinnamon roll chaffle:</u>

- 1 cup finely shredded mozzarella cheese
- 2 eggs
- 2 tablespoons almond flour
- 2 teaspoons swerve sweetener
- ½ teaspoon baking powder
- 2 teaspoons ground cinnamon

<u>For cinnamon swirl:</u>

- 2 teaspoons confectioners' swerve
- 2 teaspoons cinnamon
- 2 tablespoons butter

<u>For cinnamon roll glaze:</u>

- 2 tablespoons butter
- ½ teaspoon vanilla extract
- 2 tablespoons cream cheese
- 4 teaspoons swerve confectioners'

**Directions:**

1. Preheat the mini waffle maker.
2. Beat eggs with a fork.
3. Add almond flour, baking powder, swerve and cinnamon into a bowl and stir. Add into the bowl of eggs. Mix until well incorporated.
4. Stir in mozzarella cheese.
5. To make cinnamon swirl: Add butter, swerve and cinnamon into a microwave safe bowl. Cook for 15 seconds. Remove from the microwave and stir until well incorporated.
6. Spoon 4 – 5 tablespoons of the batter into the waffle maker. Drizzle a tablespoon of the cinnamon swirl over the batter. Swirl lightly. Set the timer for about 4 minutes. Close the waffle maker.
7. Check after about 5 minutes. Cook until crisp.
8. Take out the chaffle and set aside on a plate. Let it sit for a couple of minutes.
9. Repeat steps 6 – 8 and make the remaining chaffles.
10. Meanwhile, to make glaze: Add butter and cream cheese into a microwave safe bowl. Cook for about 10 – 12 seconds. Whisk well. If it is not smooth, cook for a few more seconds and whisk again.

11. Stir in vanilla extract and swerve and whisk well. Brush the glaze over the chaffles and serve.

# Oreo Chaffle

Makes: 4

## Ingredients:

- 2 eggs
- 4 tablespoons Monk fruit sweetener or any other keto friendly sweetener of your choice
- 2 teaspoons coconut flour
- 1 teaspoon vanilla extract
- 3 tablespoon cocoa, unsweetened
- 2 tablespoons heavy cream
- 1 teaspoon baking powder

For filling:

- Whipped cream

## Directions:

1. Preheat the mini waffle maker.
2. Beat egg with a fork. Add vanilla and whisk well.
3. Add coconut flour, sweetener, cocoa, baking powder and heavy cream into a bowl and stir until well combined. Add into the bowl of eggs. Whisk well.

4. Spoon ¼ of the batter into the waffle maker. Set the timer for about 3 – 5 minutes. Close the waffle maker.

5. Take out the chaffle and set aside on a plate. Let it sit for a couple of minutes.

6. Repeat steps 4 – 5 and make the remaining chaffles.

7. Top with whipped cream and serve.

# Pumpkin Chocolate Chip Chaffle

Makes: 6

**Ingredients:**

- 1 cup finely shredded mozzarella cheese
- 2 large eggs
- ½ teaspoon pumpkin pie spice
- 2 tablespoons almond flour
- 8 teaspoons pumpkin puree
- 4 tablespoons granulated swerve or erythritol
- 8 teaspoons sugar-free chocolate chips

To serve:

- Whipped cream (optional)

**Directions:**

1. Preheat the mini waffle maker.
2. Beat eggs with a fork. Add pumpkin puree and whisk well.
3. Add almond flour, baking powder, erythritol and pumpkin pie spice into a bowl and stir until well combined. Add into the bowl of egg mixture. Whisk well.
4. Stir in mozzarella cheese. Add chocolate chips and stir.

5. Spoon about 1/6 of the batter into the waffle maker. Set the timer for about 4 minutes. Close the waffle maker.

6. Take out the chaffle and set aside on a plate. Let it sit for a couple of minutes.

7. Repeat steps 5 – 6 and make the remaining chaffles.

8. Top with whipped cream if desired and serve.

## Strawberry Shortcake Chaffle

Makes: 4

### Ingredients:

- 2 eggs
- 2 teaspoons coconut flour
- 1 teaspoon cake batter extract
- 2 tablespoons heavy whipping cream
- 4 tablespoons swerve or erythritol
- ½ teaspoon baking powder

To serve:

- Whipped cream
- Small strawberries
- Blueberries
- Swerve confectioners

## Directions:

1. Preheat the mini waffle maker.
2. Beat eggs with a fork.
3. Add coconut flour, cake batter extract, heavy whipping cream, erythritol and baking powder and stir until well combined.
4. Spoon about ¼ of the batter into the waffle maker. Set the timer for about 3 – 5 minutes. Close the waffle maker.
5. Take out the chaffle and set aside on a plate. Let it sit for a couple of minutes.
6. Repeat steps 4 – 5 and make the remaining chaffles.
7. Sprinkle some swerve confectioners. Scatter strawberries and blueberries on top and serve with whipped cream.

# Chocolate Chip Chaffle

Makes: 4

## Ingredients:

- 1 cup finely shredded mozzarella cheese
- 2 eggs
- 1 tablespoon granulated swerve or erythritol
- 2 tablespoons almond flour
- ½ teaspoon ground cinnamon
- ¼ cup sugar-free chocolate chips

To serve:

- Whipped cream
- Powdered swerve or erythritol

## Directions:

1. Preheat the mini waffle maker.
2. Beat eggs with a fork. Add pumpkin puree and whisk well.
3. Add almond flour, baking powder, erythritol and cinnamon into a bowl and stir until well combined. Add into the bowl of egg mixture. Whisk well.
4. Stir in mozzarella cheese. Add chocolate chips and stir.

5. Spoon about 1/6 of the batter into the waffle maker. Set the timer for about 4 minutes. Close the waffle maker.
6. Take out the chaffle and set aside on a plate. Let it sit for a couple of minutes.
7. Repeat steps 5 – 6 and make the remaining chaffles.
8. Top with whipped cream. Sprinkle powdered swerve on top and serve.

# Pumpkin Cheesecake Chaffle

Makes: 2 cheesecake chaffles

## Ingredients:

### For pumpkin chaffle:

- 1 cup finely shredded mozzarella cheese
- 2 tablespoons almond flour
- 4 teaspoons heavy cream
- ½ tablespoon pumpkin pie spice
- 1 teaspoon vanilla extract
- 3 tablespoons pumpkin puree
- 2 tablespoons lakanto golden sweetener erythritol or swerve
- 2 eggs
- 2 teaspoons cream cheese, softened
- 1 teaspoon baking powder
- 2 teaspoons sugar-free maple syrup or ½ teaspoon maple extract

### For filling:

- 4 tablespoons cream cheese
- ½ teaspoon vanilla extract

- 2 tablespoons Lakanto powdered sweetener or powdered swerve or powdered erythritol

**Directions:**

1. Preheat the mini waffle maker.
2. Beat eggs with a fork. Add vanilla, pumpkin puree, heavy cream, maple syrup, and cream cheese and whisk well.
3. Add almond flour, baking powder, erythritol and pumpkin pie spice into a bowl and stir until well combined. Add into the bowl of egg mixture. Whisk well.
4. Stir in mozzarella cheese.
5. Spoon about 4 – 5 tablespoons of the batter into the waffle maker. Set the timer for about 3 - 5 minutes. Close the waffle maker.
6. Check after about 5 minutes. Cook longer if necessary.
7. Take out the chaffle and set aside on a plate. Let it sit for a couple of minutes.
8. Repeat steps 5 – 7 and make the remaining chaffles.
9. To make filling: Add cream cheese, vanilla and powdered sweetener into a bowl and whisk well.
10. Spread the filling on 2 of the chaffles. Cover with the remaining 2 chaffles and serve.

# Double Chocolate Chaffle

Makes: 4

## Ingredients:

- 2 large eggs
- 2 tablespoons sugar-free chocolate syrup
- 2 tablespoons sweetener of your choice
- 1 teaspoon vanilla extract
- ½ teaspoon baking powder
- 1 tablespoon cocoa or cacao
- 2 ounces cream cheese, softened

To serve:

- Melted butter

## Directions:

1. Beat eggs with a fork. Add vanilla, chocolate syrup and cream cheese and whisk well.
2. Add baking powder, erythritol and cocoa into a bowl and stir until well combined. Add into the bowl of egg mixture. Whisk well.
3. Stir in mozzarella cheese.

4. Spoon about 4 – 5 tablespoons of the batter into the waffle maker. Set the timer for about 6 – 8 minutes. Close the waffle maker.
5. Check after about 5 minutes. Cook until crisp.
6. Take out the chaffle and set aside on a plate. Let it sit for a couple of minutes.
7. Repeat steps 5 – 6 and make the remaining chaffles.
8. Brush with some melted butter and serve.

# Keto Bacon Maple Chaffle

Makes: 4

## Ingredients:

- 4 eggs
- 4 tablespoons heavy cream
- 2 tablespoons sugar-free maple pecan syrup
- ½ cup almond flour
- ¼ cup chopped bacon
- 1 ½ teaspoons baking powder
- 2 – 3 tablespoons butter, chopped into small cubes + extra melted butter to serve

## Directions:

1. Preheat a regular waffle maker.
2. Beat eggs with a fork. Add maple pecan syrup and heavy cream and whisk well.
3. Add baking powder and almond flour into a bowl and stir until well combined. Add into the bowl of egg mixture. Whisk well.
4. Place a few cubes of butter in the waffle maker. Butter will melt. Brush the butter inside the waffle plates.

5. Spoon about ¼ of the batter into the waffle maker. Set the timer for about 6 minutes. Close the waffle maker.

6. Open the lid after about 2 minutes. Place some more butter cubes over the chaffle. Close the waffle maker and continue cooking until the crispness you desire is achieved.

7. Take out the chaffle and set aside on a plate. Let it sit for a couple of minutes.

8. Repeat steps 5 – 7 and make the remaining chaffles.

9. Brush with some melted butter and serve.

# Vanilla Chaffle

Makes: 2

## Ingredients:

- 1 tablespoon butter, melted
- 1 large egg
- 1 ounce cream cheese, softened
- 2 tablespoons lakanto confectioners'
- 1 tablespoon coconut flour
- 2 tablespoons almond flour
- ¼ teaspoon vanilla cupcake extract
- ½ teaspoon vanilla extract
- A pinch Himalayan pink salt
- ½ teaspoon baking powder

## Directions:

1. Preheat the mini waffle maker.
2. Cool the melted butter to room temperature.
3. Beat eggs with a fork. Add melted butter and cream cheese and whisk well. Add vanilla, vanilla cupcake extract, salt and lakanto and whisk well.

4. Add almond flour, baking powder and coconut flour into a bowl and stir until well combined. Add into the bowl of eggs. Stir until well combined.
5. Pour ½ the batter into the waffle maker. Set the timer for about 4 minutes. Close the waffle maker.
6. Check after about 4 minutes. Cook further if required.
7. Take out the chaffle and set aside on a plate. Let it sit for a couple of minutes.
8. Repeat steps 5 – 7 and make the remaining chaffle.

# Cinnamon Chaffles

Makes: 4 chaffles

**Ingredients:**

**Ingredients:**

- 1 cups finely shredded mozzarella cheese
- 2 tablespoons vanilla extract
- 2 tablespoons almond flour
- 
- 2 eggs
- 2 teaspoons baking powder
- ½ teaspoon ground cinnamon

To serve:

- Melted butter
- Sugar-free syrup
- Ground cinnamon

**Directions:**

1. Preheat the mini waffle maker.
2. Beat eggs with a fork. Add vanilla and whisk well.

3. Add almond flour, baking powder and cinnamon into a bowl and stir until well combined. Add into the bowl of eggs. Stir until well combined.
4. Stir in mozzarella cheese.
5. Spoon ¼ of the batter into the waffle maker. Set the timer for about 10 minutes. Close the waffle maker.
6. Check after about 5 minutes. Cook until crisp.
7. Take out the chaffle when cooked and set aside on a plate. Let it sit for a couple of minutes.
8. Repeat steps 5 – 6 and make the remaining chaffles.
9. Brush with some melted butter. Drizzle some sugar-free syrup on top. Garnish with ground cinnamon and serve.

# Keto S'mores Chaffle

Makes: 4

## Ingredients:

- 1 cup finely shredded mozzarella cheese
- 2 large eggs
- 4 tablespoons swerve sweetener, brown
- ½ teaspoon baking powder
- 1 teaspoon psyllium husk powder
- 1/8 teaspoon Himalayan pink salt
- 4 tablespoons keto marshmallow crème fluff
- 1 teaspoon vanilla extract
- ½ Lily's original dark chocolate bar, shredded

<u>For marshmallow crème fluff:</u>

- 2 tablespoons heavy whipping cream, very chilled
- ¼ teaspoon pure vanilla extract
- ¼ teaspoon xanthan gum
- 2 tablespoons swerve confectioners'
- 1/8 teaspoon Himalayan pink salt

## Directions:

1. To make marshmallow crème fluff: Add sweetener into a bowl. Add cream over the sweetener. Add vanilla and Himalayan pink salt. Beat with an electric hand mixer until it fluffs up. Add a wee bit of the xanthan gum and fold gently with a spatula. Continue adding a wee bit of xanthan gum and fold gently each time. Chill until use.

2. Preheat the mini waffle maker.

3. Beat eggs with a fork. Add vanilla and whisk well.

4. Add swerve sweetener, Himalayan pink salt, baking powder and psyllium husk powder into a bowl and stir until well combined. Add into the bowl of eggs. Whisk well.

5. Stir in mozzarella cheese. Let the batter sit for 5 minutes.

6. Spoon ¼ of the batter into the waffle maker. Set the timer for about 3 – 4 minutes. Close the waffle maker.

7. Check after about 4 minutes. Cook for some more time if necessary.

8. Take out the chaffle and set aside on a plate. Let it sit for a couple of minutes.

9. Repeat steps 6 – 8 and make the remaining chaffles.

10. Top with marshmallow crème fluff and serve.

# Banana Nut Chaffle

Makes: 4

**Ingredients:**

- 2 eggs
- 2 tablespoons sugar-free cheesecake pudding mix (optional)
- 2 tablespoons cream cheese, softened, at room temperature
- 2 tablespoons Monk fruit confectioners'
- ½ teaspoon banana extract
- ½ teaspoon vanilla extract
- 1 cup shredded mozzarella cheese

To serve: Optional

- Chopped pecans
- Sugar-free caramel sauce

**Directions:**

1. Preheat the mini waffle maker.
2. Beat eggs with a fork. Add vanilla, cream cheese, mozzarella cheese, banana extract and monk fruit sweetener and whisk well.

3. Pour ¼ of the batter into the waffle maker. Set the timer for about 4 minutes. Close the waffle maker.
4. Check after about 4 minutes. Cook further if required.
5. Take out the chaffle and set aside on a plate. Let it sit for a couple of minutes.
6. Repeat steps 3 – 5 and make the remaining chaffle.
7. Drizzle caramel sauce on top. Sprinkle pecans and serve.

# Keto Peanut Butter Cup Chaffle

Makes: 4 (2 servings)

## Ingredients:

<u>For chaffle:</u>

- 2 tablespoons heavy cream
- 2 tablespoons lakanto golden sweetener erythritol or swerve
- 1 teaspoon vanilla extract
- 2 eggs
- 2 teaspoons coconut flour
- 2 tablespoons unsweetened cocoa
- 1 teaspoon baking powder
- 1 teaspoon cake batter flavor extract

<u>For filling:</u>

- 6 tablespoons natural peanut butter
- 4 tablespoons heavy cream
- 4 teaspoons lakanto powdered sweetener

## Directions:

1. Preheat the mini waffle maker.

2. Beat eggs with a fork. Add vanilla, heavy cream, sweetener, vanilla, coconut flour, cocoa, baking powder and cake batter flavor extract and whisk well. Let the batter sit for 3 to 4 minutes.

3. Pour ¼ of the batter into the waffle maker. Set the timer for about 4 minutes. Close the waffle maker.

4. Check after about 4 minutes. Cook further if required.

5. Take out the chaffle and set aside on a plate. Let it sit for a couple of minutes.

6. Repeat steps 3 – 5 and make the remaining chaffles.

7. To make peanut butter filling: Add peanut butter, cream and sweetener into a bowl and whisk well.

8. Spread peanut butter filling over 2 of the chaffles. Cover with the remaining 2 chaffles and serve.

# Apple Pie Chaffles

Makes: 2

## Ingredients:

- 2 1/3 cups finely shredded mozzarella cheese
- 2 tablespoons sugar-free chocolate chips
- 2 large eggs
- 1 teaspoon apple pie spice

<u>To serve:</u>

- Butter

## Directions:

1. Preheat the regular waffle maker.
2. Beat eggs with a fork.
3. Sprinkle half the cheese in the waffle maker.
4. Pour half the eggs over it. Sprinkle half the apple pie spice and half the chocolate chips on top.
5. Set the timer for about 4 minutes. Close the waffle maker.
6. Check after about 4 minutes. Cook further if required.
7. Take out the chaffle and set aside on a plate. Let it sit for a couple of minutes.
8. Repeat steps 4 – 7 and make the remaining chaffles.
9. Top with butter and serve.

# Krispy Kreme Copycat Glazed Raspberry Jelly-Filled Donut Chaffle

Makes: 4 chaffle donuts

**Ingredients:**

<u>For chaffles:</u>

- ½ cup shredded mozzarella cheese
- 2 tablespoons swerve or erythritol
- 2 large eggs
- 4 tablespoons cream cheese, softened
- 1 teaspoon baking powder
- 2 tablespoons almond flour
- 40 drops glazed donut flavoring

<u>For raspberry jelly filling:</u>

- ½ cup raspberries
- 2 teaspoons swerve confectioners
- 2 teaspoons chia seeds

<u>For donut glaze:</u>

- ¼ teaspoon water or heavy cream
- 2 teaspoons swerve confectioners

**Directions:**

1. Preheat the mini waffle maker.
2. Beat eggs with a fork. Add cream cheese and whisk well.
3. Add almond flour, baking powder and sweetener into a bowl and stir until well combined. Add into the bowl of egg mixture. Mix until well combined.
4. Stir in mozzarella cheese and donut flavoring.
5. Spoon about 4 – 5 tablespoons of the batter into the waffle maker. Set the timer for about 2 - 3 minutes. Close the waffle maker.
6. Check after about 3 minutes. Cook further if required.
7. Take out the chaffle and set aside on a plate. Let it sit for a couple of minutes.
8. Repeat steps 5 – 6 and make the remaining chaffles.
9. Meanwhile make the raspberry jelly filling as follows: Add raspberries, sweetener and chia seeds into a saucepan. Place the saucepan over medium heat. Simmer until raspberries are cooked. Mash it simultaneously as it cooks.
10. To make donut glaze: Mix together sweetener and water in a bowl.
11. Place 2 chaffles on a serving plate. Divide the raspberry jam and spread over the chaffles.
12. Cover with the remaining 2 chaffles. Drizzle the glaze on top and serve.

# Gingerbread Cookies Chaffle with Maple Icing

Makes: 4 chaffles

**Ingredients:**

For chaffle:

- 2 eggs
- 4 teaspoons butter, melted
- 4 teaspoon coconut flour
- 2 tablespoons almond flour
- ½ teaspoon baking powder
- 1 teaspoon ground ginger
- ¼ teaspoon ground cloves
- 1 ½ teaspoons ground ginger
- ¼ teaspoon ground nutmeg
- 2 ounces cream cheese, softened
- 2 tablespoons swerve brown sweetener

For maple icing:

- 4 tablespoons powdered swerve or any other keto friendly sweetener of your choice
- ¼ teaspoon maple extract
- 3 teaspoons heavy cream
- 1 teaspoon water or more if required

- Ground cinnamon, to garnish

## Directions:

1. Preheat the mini waffle maker.
2. Cool the melted butter to room temperature.
3. Beat eggs with a fork. Add melted butter and cream cheese whisk well.
4. Add almond flour, spices, baking powder and coconut flour into a bowl and stir until well combined. Add into the bowl of eggs. Stir until well combined.
5. Pour ¼ of the batter into the waffle maker. Set the timer for about 4 minutes. Close the waffle maker.
6. Check after about 4 minutes. Cook further if required.
7. Take out the chaffle and set aside on a plate. Let it sit for a couple of minutes.
8. Repeat steps 5 – 7 and make the remaining chaffles.
9. To make icing: Add sweetener, maple extract and heavy cream into a bowl and whisk well. Add water if the mixture is very thick.
10. Spoon the icing over the chaffles. Garnish with cinnamon and serve.

# Bread Pudding

Serves: 2 – 3

For chaffles:

- 1 tablespoon butter, melted
- 1 large egg
- 1 ounce cream cheese, softened
- 2 tablespoons Monk fruit sweetener
- 1 tablespoon coconut flour
- 2 tablespoons almond flour
- ½ teaspoon baking powder
- ½ teaspoon vanilla extract

Other ingredients:

- 2 tablespoons butter, melted
- 1 egg
- 3 – 4 tablespoons swerve or splenda
- 2 teaspoons vanilla extract
- ¼ teaspoon ground nutmeg
- ½ teaspoon ground cinnamon
- 1 ¼ cups lukewarm milk of your choice

**Directions:**

1. Preheat the mini waffle maker.

2. Cool the melted butter to room temperature.

3. Beat eggs with a fork. Add melted butter and cream cheese and whisk well. Add vanilla, vanilla cupcake extract, salt and lakanto and whisk well.

4. Add almond flour, baking powder and coconut flour into a bowl and stir until well combined. Add into the bowl of eggs. Stir until well combined.

5. Pour ½ of the batter into the waffle maker. Set the timer for about 4 minutes. Close the waffle maker.

6. Check after about 4 minutes. Cook further if required.

7. Take out the chaffle and set aside on a plate.

8. Repeat steps 5 – 7 and make the remaining chaffle. Let the chaffles cool completely. Chop or tear into bite size pieces.

9. Place chaffle pieces in a baking dish.

10. Add egg, milk, butter, sweetener, vanilla, nutmeg and cinnamon into a bowl and whisk well. Drizzle over the chaffles. Stir to coat.

11. Bake in a preheated oven at 350°F for about 30 minutes.

12. Remove from the oven and cool for a few minutes before serving.

13. Serve with whipped cream or heavy cream.

# Pumpkin Pecan Chaffle

Makes: 4 chaffles

## Ingredients:

- 1 cup finely shredded mozzarella cheese
- ½ tablespoon pumpkin pie spice
- 2 teaspoons erythritol
- 2 eggs
- 2 tablespoons pumpkin puree
- ¼ cup chopped pecans, lightly toasted
- 4 tablespoons almond flour

To serve:

- Pecans, chopped, toasted
- Sugar-free caramel syrup

## Directions:

1. Preheat the mini waffle maker.
2. Beat eggs with a fork. Add pumpkin puree and whisk well.
3. Add almond flour, erythritol and pumpkin pie spice and stir until well combined. Add into the bowl of egg mixture. Mix until well combined.
4. Stir in mozzarella cheese and pecans.

5. Spoon ¼ of the batter into the waffle maker. Set the timer for about 5 minutes. Close the waffle maker.
6. Check after about 5 minutes. Cook for longer if required.
7. Take out the chaffle and set aside on a plate. Let it sit for a couple of minutes.
8. Repeat steps 5 – 6 and make the remaining chaffles.
9. Brush with some melted butter and serve topped with sugar-free caramel sauce and pecans.

# Protein Vanilla Chaffles

Makes: 2 chaffles

## Ingredients:

- ¼ cup finely shredded mozzarella cheese
- 1 large egg
- ¼ scoop keto friendly protein powder
- ½ tablespoon sweetener
- 1 teaspoon vanilla extract

## Directions:

1. Preheat the mini waffle maker.
2. Beat egg with a fork. Add vanilla and whisk well.
3. Add protein powder and stir until well combined.
4. Stir in mozzarella cheese.
5. Spoon ½ the batter into the waffle maker. Set the timer for about 5 minutes. Close the waffle maker.
6. Check after about 5 minutes. Cook for longer if you prefer it to be crisp.
7. Take out the chaffle when cooked and set aside on a plate. Let it sit for a couple of minutes.
8. Repeat steps 5 – 6 and make the remaining chaffles.

# Raspberry Almond Chaffles

Makes: 2

## Ingredients:

For chaffles:

- ½ cup shredded mozzarella cheese
- 2 tablespoons swerve or erythritol
- 2 large eggs
- 4 tablespoons almond flour
- 2 tablespoons swerve confectioners
- 1 teaspoon almond extract, divided
- 4 tablespoons heavy cream
- 2/3 cup raspberries, divided
- 2 ounces cream cheese, softened
- ½ teaspoon baking powder
- 1/8 teaspoon salt
- 2 teaspoons Sukrin gold fiber syrup or any other sugar-free sweetener of your choice

## Directions:

1. Preheat the mini waffle maker.

2. Add eggs, almond flour, baking powder, sweetener, ¼ cup raspberries, cream cheese and ½ teaspoon almond extract into a blender and blend until smooth.

3. Spoon ½ the batter into the waffle maker. Set the timer for about 2 - 3 minutes. Close the waffle maker.

4. Check after about 3 minutes. Cook further if required.

5. Take out the chaffle and set aside on a plate. Let it sit for a couple of minutes.

6. Repeat steps 3 – 5 and make the remaining chaffles.

7. In the meantime, add heavy cream, ½ teaspoon almond extract and sweetener into a bowl. Beat with an electric hand mixer until soft peaks are formed.

8. Place chaffles on a serving platter. Divide the cream among the chaffles and spread over the chaffles. Scatter rest of the raspberries on top and serve.

# Cinnamon Swirl Chaffles

Makes: 4

## Ingredients:

- 2 ounces cream cheese, softened
- 2 teaspoons vanilla extract
- 2 tablespoons splenda
- 2 eggs
- 2 tablespoons very fine almond flour
- 2 teaspoons ground cinnamon

For icing:

- 2 tablespoons unsalted butter
- 1 teaspoon vanilla extract
- 2 ounces cream cheese
- 2 tablespoons splenda

For cinnamon drizzle:

- 1 tablespoon butter
- 2 teaspoons ground cinnamon
- 2 tablespoons splenda

## Directions:

1. Preheat the mini waffle maker.
2. Beat eggs with a fork. Add vanilla and cream cheese and whisk well.
3. Add almond flour, splenda and cinnamon into a bowl and stir until well combined. Add into the bowl of eggs. Stir until well combined.
4. Spoon ¼ of the batter into the waffle maker. Set the timer for about 5 – 6 minutes. Close the waffle maker.
5. Check after about 5 minutes. Cook until crisp.
6. Take out the chaffle when cooked and set aside on a plate. Let it sit for a couple of minutes.
7. Repeat steps 4 – 6 and make the remaining chaffles.
8. To make cinnamon drizzle: Add cinnamon, butter and splenda into a microwave safe bowl. Microwave on high for 10 seconds. Mix well.
9. To make icing: Add butter, vanilla, cream cheese and splenda into a bowl and whisk well.
10. Place the chaffles on a serving platter. Spread the icing over the chaffles. Trickle the cinnamon swirl over the icing. Swirl lightly with a toothpick.
11. Serve.

# Chaffle French Toast Sticks

Makes: 8 sticks

## Ingredients:

- 3 eggs
- 2 tablespoons coconut flour
- ½ teaspoon ground cinnamon
- 1 cup shredded mozzarella cheese
- 4 tablespoons powdered swerve
- 4 tablespoons butter

## Directions:

1. Add 2 eggs into a bowl and beat well.
2. Stir in mozzarella cheese, swerve, coconut flour and ¼ teaspoon cinnamon. Stir until well incorporated.
3. Preheat the regular waffle maker.
4. Spoon ½ the batter into the waffle maker. Set the timer for about 6 – 8 minutes. Close the waffle maker.
5. Check after about 5 minutes. Cook until crisp.
6. Take out the chaffle when cooked and set aside on a plate. Let it sit for a couple of minutes.
7. Repeat steps 4 – 6 and make the other chaffle.
8. Place the chaffles on your cutting board. Cut each into 4 strips.

9. Beat the 3<sup>rd</sup> egg along with ¼ teaspoon cinnamon. Dip the sticks in the egg mixture, one at a time and shake to drop off excess egg.

10. Place on a baking sheet lined with aluminum foil. Also brush the aluminum foil with butter.

11. Bake in a preheated oven at 375°F for about 20 minutes. Brush some butter on the sticks after about 8 – 10 minutes of baking. Flip sides after brushing with butter. Bake until golden brown.

# Overnight French Toast Casserole

Makes: 6 servings

**Ingredients:**

For chaffles:

- 1 tablespoon butter, melted
- 1 large egg
- 1 ounce cream cheese, softened
- 2 tablespoons lakanto confectioners
- 1 tablespoon coconut flour
- 2 tablespoons almond flour
- ½ teaspoon baking powder
- ½ teaspoon vanilla extract
- A pinch Himalayan pink salt

Other ingredients:

- 2 eggs, beaten
- ¼ cup swerve or sukrin gold
- ¼ cup heavy whipping cream
- ½ teaspoon ground cinnamon

For topping:

- ½ cup chopped pecans

- 1 tablespoon sukrin gold
- 3 tablespoons butter, melted

**Directions:**

1. Preheat the mini waffle maker.
2. Cool the melted butter to room temperature.
3. Beat eggs with a fork. Add melted butter and cream cheese and whisk well. Add vanilla, vanilla cupcake extract, salt and lakanto and whisk well.
4. Add almond flour, baking powder and coconut flour into a bowl and stir until well combined. Add into the bowl of eggs. Stir until well combined.
5. Pour ½ of the batter into the waffle maker. Set the timer for about 4 minutes. Close the waffle maker.
6. Check after about 4 minutes. Cook further if required.
7. Take out the chaffle and set aside on a plate.
8. Repeat steps 5 – 7 and make the remaining chaffle. Let the chaffles cool completely. Chop or tear into bite size pieces.
9. Place chaffle pieces in a baking dish or casserole dish.
10. Add eggs, sukrin gold, whipping cream and cinnamon into a bowl and whisk well. Drizzle over the chaffles. Stir to coat. Chill overnight.
11. Remove from the refrigerator 30 minutes before baking.

12. To make topping: Add butter, sukrin gold and pecans into a bowl and mix well. Scatter on top of the casserole.
13. Bake in a preheated oven at 350°F for about 30 minutes.
14. Remove from the oven and cool for a few minutes before serving.

# Blueberry Chaffle Pudding

Makes: 3

## Ingredients:

- ½ cup finely shredded mozzarella cheese
- 1 egg
- 1 tablespoon almond flour
- 1 teaspoon swerve sweetener
- ½ teaspoon baking powder
- ½ teaspoon ground cinnamon
- 1 ½ tablespoons fresh blueberries

Other ingredients:

- 1 cup almond milk
- ½ teaspoon vanilla extract
- ½ teaspoon ground cinnamon
- 3 large eggs
- ½ teaspoon swerve sweetener
- ½ cup frozen blueberries

## Directions:

1. Preheat the mini waffle maker.
2. Beat egg with a fork. Add vanilla and whisk well.

3. Add almond flour, baking powder, swerve and cinnamon into a bowl and stir until well combined. Add into the bowl of eggs. Mix well.
4. Stir in mozzarella cheese and blueberries.
5. Pour 1/3 of the batter into the waffle maker. Set the timer for 4 minutes. Close the waffle maker.
6. Take out the chaffle and set aside on a plate. Let it sit for a couple of minutes.
7. Repeat steps 5 – 6 and make the remaining chaffles. When cool enough to handle, cut or chop the chaffles.
8. Place the chaffle pieces in a baking dish.
9. Add almond milk, vanilla, cinnamon, eggs and sweetener into a bowl and whisk well. Pour over the chaffle pieces. Stir until well combined.
10. Scatter blueberries and stir until well combined.
11. Bake in a preheated oven at 350°F for about 30 minutes.

## Chocolate Brownie Chaffles

Makes: 10 – 12 chaffles

**Ingredients:**

- 1 cup sugar-free chocolate chips

- 6 eggs
- 2 teaspoons vanilla extract
- 1 cup butter
- ½ cup Truvia or any other keto friendly sweetener of your choice

**Directions:**

1. Add butter and chocolate into a microwave safe bowl. Microwave on high for a minute. Whisk well.
2. Add eggs, vanilla and truvia into a bowl and whisk well.
3. Add melted chocolate in a thin drizzle, beating simultaneously until well combined.
4. Preheat a mini waffle maker.
5. Pour about 3 tablespoons of the batter into the waffle maker. Set the timer for 4 minutes. Close the waffle maker.
6. Take out the chaffle and set aside on a plate. Let it sit for a couple of minutes.
7. Repeat steps 5 – 6 and make the remaining chaffles

# Mint and Chocolate Chaffles

Makes: 10 – 12 chaffles

## Ingredients:

- 1 cup sugar-free chocolate chips
- 6 eggs
- 2 teaspoons vanilla extract
- ¼ teaspoon mint extract
- 1 cup butter
- ½ cup Truvia or any other keto friendly sweetener of your choice
- ¼ cup chopped pecans

For maple pecan butter cream frosting:

- ¼ cup chopped pecans
- 2 ounces cream cheese, softened
- 2 tablespoons heavy whipping cream
- 2 ounces butter
- ¼ cup powdered swerve
- 1 teaspoon maple extract

## Directions:

1. Add butter and chocolate into a microwave safe bowl. Microwave on high for a minute. Whisk well.
2. Add eggs, vanilla, mint extract and truvia into a bowl and whisk well.
3. Add melted chocolate in a thin drizzle, beating simultaneously until well combined.
4. Stir in the pecans.
5. Preheat a mini waffle maker.
6. Pour about 3 tablespoons of the batter into the waffle maker. Set the timer for 4 minutes. Close the waffle maker.
7. Take out the chaffle and set aside on a plate. Let it sit for a couple of minutes. Repeat steps 6 – 7 and make the remaining chaffles.
8. To make maple pecan butter cream frosting: Add pecans, cream cheese, cream, butter, swerve and maple extract into a blender and blend until smooth.
9. Spread over the chaffles and serve.

# Chapter 2: Keto Chicken Chaffle Recipes

## Easy Chicken Parmesan Chaffle

Makes: 4 chaffles

**Ingredients:**

For chaffle:

- 1 cup canned or cooked, shredded chicken
- ¼ cup shredded Parmesan cheese
- ½ cup shredded cheddar cheese
- 2 eggs
- ¼ teaspoon garlic powder
- 2 teaspoons Italian seasoning + extra to serve
- 2 teaspoons cream cheese, at room temperature

For topping:

- 2 tablespoons keto friendly pizza sauce
- 4 slices provolone cheese

**Directions:**

1. Plug on the mini waffle maker and allow it to preheat.

2. Add chicken, cheddar cheese, Parmesan cheese, eggs, garlic powder, Italian seasoning and cream cheese into a bowl and whisk well.
3. Scatter a little cheese (apart from what is mentioned in the recipe), preferably mozzarella cheese on the waffle maker initially.
4. Close the lid and let it cook for half a minute.
5. Next pour ¼ of the egg mixture. Sprinkle some more cheese over the egg mixture if desired.
6. Set the timer for 4 – 6 minutes. Check after about 4 to 5 minutes. Cook for a few more minutes if it looks uncooked.
7. Remove onto a plate and let it cool for a couple of minutes. Spread some pizza sauce on top. Place a slice of provolone cheese on top. Sprinkle some Italian seasoning on top and serve.
8. Repeat steps 3 – 7 and make the remaining chaffles.

# BBQ Chicken Chaffle

Makes: 4 chaffles

## Ingredients:

<u>For chaffle:</u>

- 2/3 cup canned or cooked, diced chicken
- 2 tablespoons sugar-free BBQ sauce + extra to serve
- 2 tablespoons almond flour
- ¼ cup shredded cheddar cheese
- 2 eggs

## Directions:

1. Preheat the mini waffle maker.
2. Beat eggs with a fork. Add BBQ sauce and almond flour and beat until well incorporated.
3. Add chicken and cheddar cheese and mix well.
4. Pour ¼ of the batter into the waffle maker. Set the timer for about 4 minutes. Close the waffle maker.
5. Check after about 4 minutes. Cook further if required.
6. Take out the chaffle and set aside on a plate. Let it sit for a couple of minutes.
7. Repeat steps 4 – 6 and make the remaining chaffle.
8. Serve with some extra sugar-free BBQ sauce.

# Jamaican Jerk Chicken Chaffle

Makes: 4 – 5

**Ingredients:**

<u>For filling:</u>

- 2 pounds ground chicken or left over chicken, finely chopped
- 1 medium onion, chopped
- 2 teaspoons dried thyme
- 4 teaspoons dried parsley
- 4 teaspoons Jerk seasoning hot and spicy
- 4 tablespoons butter
- 2 teaspoons granulated garlic
- ¼ teaspoon pepper
- 1 ½ teaspoons salt or to taste
- 1 chicken broth
- 1 tablespoon butter

<u>For chaffle:</u>

- 2 tablespoons butter, melted
- 2 eggs
- 4 tablespoons almond flour
- ½ teaspoon baking powder

- 1 cup finely shredded mozzarella cheese
- 1/8 teaspoon xanthan gum
- ¼ teaspoon garlic powder
- ½ teaspoon turmeric powder
- ¼ teaspoon onion powder
- A large pinch salt

**Directions:**

1. To make filling: Place a skillet over medium heat. Add butter. When butter melts, add onion and sauté until translucent.
2. Stir in thyme, parsley and jerk seasoning. Sauté for a few seconds until aromatic.
3. Add chicken and broth. Mix well. When it begins to boil, lower the heat and cook for about 10 – 15 minutes. Increase the heat to high heat and cook until dry. Turn off the heat. Cover and keep warm.
4. To make chaffles: Preheat the mini waffle maker.
5. Cool the melted butter to room temperature.
6. Beat eggs with a fork. Add melted butter and whisk well. Add salt, turmeric powder, onion powder and garlic powder and whisk well.

7.  Add almond flour and baking powder into a bowl and stir until well combined. Add into the bowl of eggs. Stir until well combined.

8.  Add mozzarella cheese and xanthan gum and stir. Let the batter sit for 5 minutes.

9.  Pour ¼ of the batter into the waffle maker. Set the timer for about 4 minutes. Close the waffle maker.

10. Check after about 4 minutes. Cook further if required.

11. Upturn a muffin tin. Take out the chaffle and place in the tin, in the gap between the cups. Let it cool completely. It will take the shape like a bowl.

12. Repeat steps 9 – 11 and make the remaining chaffles.

13. Place the filling in the tacos and serve.

# Amish Style Chicken Chaffle

Makes: 4 chaffles

## Ingredients:

- 1 cup grated cheddar cheese
- 2 eggs
- 2 teaspoons baking powder
- 4 tablespoons blanched almond flour

### For chicken and gravy:

- 1 cup cooked, coarsely shredded chicken breast
- 4 tablespoons blanched almond flour
- 6 tablespoons heavy cream
- ¼ teaspoon pepper or to taste
- Salt to taste
- 1 teaspoon xanthan gum
- 4 tablespoons unsalted butter, melted
- 2 cups chicken stock
- ¼ teaspoon ground poultry seasoning
- 2 scallions, sliced

## Directions:

1. To make chicken and gravy: Place a skillet over medium heat. Add butter. When butter melts, add almond flour. Whisk well.

2. Cook until light brown. Add chicken stock, stirring constantly. Stir in heavy cream, xanthan gum, poultry seasoning, pepper and salt. Simmer until thick. Stir occasionally. Turn off the heat. Cover and keep warm.

3. Preheat the mini waffle maker.

4. Beat eggs with a fork. Stir in cheddar cheese and almond flour.

5. Spoon ¼ of the batter into the waffle maker. Set the timer for 3- 4 minutes. Close the waffle maker.

6. Take out the chaffle when cooked and set aside on a plate. Let it sit for a couple of minutes.

7. Repeat steps 5 – 6 and make the remaining chaffles.

8. Serve chaffles with chicken and gravy. Garnish with scallions and serve.

## Savory Buffalo Chicken Chaffle

Makes: 4 chaffles

**Ingredients:**

- 10 ounces canned or cooked chicken

- 10 tablespoons shredded cheddar cheese
- 2 eggs
- 4 tablespoons buffalo sauce
- 4 ounces cream cheese, softened

## Directions:

1. Beat eggs with a fork. Stir in cheddar cheese, chicken, cream cheese, buffalo and sauce.
2. Scatter some mozzarella cheese on the bottom of the waffle maker.
3. Spoon ¼ of the batter into the waffle maker. Set the timer for 3- 5 minutes. Scatter some mozzarella cheese on top of the batter. Close the waffle maker. Check after about 4 minutes. Cook further if you desire a crisp chaffle.
4. Take out the chaffle when cooked and set aside on a plate. Let it sit for a couple of minutes.
5. Repeat steps 3 – 4 and make the remaining chaffles.

# Chick Fila Copycat Chaffle Sandwich

Makes: 4 chaffles (2 sandwiches)

**Ingredients:**

For chicken:

- 2 chicken breasts
- 4 tablespoons powdered Parmesan cheese
- 2 teaspoons ground flaxseeds
- 4 tablespoons butter, melted
- ½ cup dill pickle juice
- 4 tablespoons ground pork rinds
- Salt to taste
- Pepper to taste

For chaffle:

- 2 cups finely shredded mozzarella cheese
- 2 eggs
- ½ teaspoon butter extract
- 6 – 10 drops stevia Glycerite

**Directions:**

1.  For chicken: Place the chicken breasts on your countertop. Pound with a meat mallet until ½ inch thick. Cut each into 2 halves.
2.  Place the chicken in a large Ziploc bag. Pour pickle juice. Seal the bag and turn the bag around a few times so that the chicken is well coated with the juice.
3.  Cook in a preheated air fryer or an oven at 400°F for about 8 to 10 minutes or until cooked through.
4.  Preheat the mini waffle maker.
5.  Beat eggs with a fork. Add butter extract and stevia Glycerite. Whisk well. Stir in the mozzarella.
6.  Spoon ¼ of the batter into the waffle maker. Set the timer for 2 to 3 minutes. Close the waffle maker.
7.  Take out the chaffle when cooked and set aside on a plate. Let it sit for a couple of minutes.
8.  Repeat steps 6 – 7 and make the remaining chaffles.
9.  Place 2 chaffles on a serving platter. Place one piece of chicken on each chaffle. Cover with the remaining chaffles and serve.

# Chaffle Sandwich

Makes: 2 chaffles (1 sandwich)

**Ingredients:**

For chaffle:

- ½ cup finely shredded mozzarella or cheddar cheese
- 1 large egg
- 2 tablespoons superfine, blanched almond flour
- ¼ teaspoon + 1/8 teaspoon baking powder
- ¼ teaspoon garlic powder

For sandwich filling: Use any

- Cooked chicken or turkey slices
- Keto chicken salad
- Bacon slices
- Keto tuna salad

**Directions:**

1. Preheat the mini waffle maker.
2. Beat eggs with a fork.
3. Add almond flour, baking powder and garlic powder into a bowl and stir until well combined. Add into the bowl of eggs. Stir until well combined.

4. Stir in mozzarella cheese.

5. Spoon ½ the batter into the waffle maker. Set the timer for about 10 minutes. Close the waffle maker.

6. Check after about 5 minutes. Cook until crisp.

7. Take out the chaffle when cooked and set aside on a plate. Let it sit for a couple of minutes.

8. Repeat steps 5 – 7 and make the remaining chaffles.

9. Place the fillings between the 2 chaffles and serve.

# Green Chili Chicken Chaffle Sandwich

Makes: 2 sandwiches

## Ingredients:

For chaffles:

- 1 cup finely shredded Mexican cheese
- 2 large eggs
- 3 tablespoons diced, canned green chilies

For chicken:

- ¼ cup aioli sauce
- 1 cup spring lettuce
- 2 chicken breasts
- 1 tablespoon olive oil

## Directions:

1. Preheat the mini waffle maker.
2. Beat eggs with a fork. Stir in the mozzarella.
3. Spoon ¼ of the batter into the waffle maker. Set the timer for 2 to 3 minutes. Close the waffle maker.
4. Take out the chaffle and set aside on a plate. Let it sit for a couple of minutes.
5. Repeat steps 3 – 4 and make the remaining chaffles.

6. Meanwhile, make the chicken as follows: Place a nonstick skillet over medium heat. Add oil. When the oil is heated, add chicken and cook until brown on both the sides and cooked through.

7. Place 2 chaffles on a serving platter. Place a chicken on each. Drizzle aioli sauce on top. Top with lettuce. Cover with the remaining chaffles and serve.

# Chicken Chaffle

Makes: 4

## Ingredients:

For chaffles:

- 1 cup grated cheddar cheese
- 2 eggs
- 2 teaspoons baking powder
- 4 tablespoons blanched almond flour
- 2 ounces cream cheese
- 1 tablespoon coconut flour
- 1 teaspoon granulated swerve
- 1 teaspoon baking powder
- ½ tablespoon psyllium husk powder

For chicken:

- Coconut oil or avocado oil, to fry
- ½ pound chicken tenderloins, lightly pounded with a meat mallet until flat, rinsed, dried with paper towels

For chicken marinade:

- ½ cup heavy whipping cream
- ½ tablespoon apple cider vinegar

- ½ teaspoon salt or to taste
- 4 teaspoons Tabasco hot sauce
- Pepper to taste

For breading chicken:

- ¼ cup fine almond flour, sifted
- 2 tablespoons finely grated Parmesan cheese
- 2 tablespoons coconut flour
- ½ teaspoon paprika
- ¼ teaspoon cayenne pepper or to taste
- ¼ teaspoon onion powder
- ¼ teaspoon garlic powder
- ½ teaspoon salt
- Pepper to taste
- 1 large egg, beaten

For cayenne maple syrup:

- 6 tablespoons sugar-free maple syrup
- 2 tablespoons cold, unsalted butter
- ½ teaspoon Tabasco sauce

**Directions:**

1. To make fried chicken: Firstly prepare the marinade by mixing together heavy cream, vinegar, salt, hot sauce and pepper in a bowl.
2. Place chicken and turn the chicken around to coat it well with the marinade. Chill for 2 – 8 hours.
3. For breading: Add almond flour, Parmesan cheese, coconut flour, paprika, cayenne pepper, onion powder, garlic powder, salt and pepper into a bowl and stir.
4. First dip the chicken in egg, one at a time. Shake to drop off excess egg. Next dredge in the flour mixture. Shake to drop off excess mixture. Place on a plate.
5. Place a pan over medium-high heat. Add oil. When the oil is heated, place chicken and cook until the underside is light brown. Flip sides and cook the other side until light brown.
6. Remove with a slotted spoon and place on a baking sheet. Cover the baking sheet lightly with foil.
7. Bake in a preheated oven at 375° F for about 20 minutes or until cooked though.
8. Meanwhile make the chaffles as follows: Preheat the mini waffle maker.
10. Beat eggs with a fork. Add cream cheese and whisk well.
11. Add almond flour, baking powder, psyllium husk powder, coconut flour and sweetener into a bowl and stir until well

combined. Add into the bowl of eggs. Stir until well combined.

12. Stir in cheddar cheese.

13. Preheat the mini waffle maker.

14. Spoon ¼ of the batter into the waffle maker. Set the timer for about 10 minutes. Close the waffle maker.

15. Check after about 5 minutes. Cook until crisp.

16. Take out the chaffle when cooked and set aside on a plate. Let it sit for a couple of minutes.

17. Repeat steps 14 – 16 and make the remaining chaffles.

18. To make cayenne maple syrup: Add maple syrup into a small saucepan. Place the saucepan over medium low heat. When it begins to bubble, add Tabasco sauce and stir. Remove from heat.

19. Add butter and stir.

20. Place chaffles on a serving platter. Place chicken on top. Drizzle cayenne maple syrup on top and serve.

# Chicken Bacon Ranch Chaffle

Makes: 4

**Ingredients:**

- 2 eggs
- ¼ cup cooked, crumbled bacon
- 2 teaspoons powdered ranch dressing
- 2/3 cup cooked, diced chicken
- 2/3 cup shredded Monterey Jack cheese

**Directions:**

1. Add eggs, cheese and ranch dressing into a bowl and whisk well.
2. Stir in the chicken and bacon.
3. Preheat the mini waffle maker.
4. Spoon ¼ of the batter into the waffle maker. Set the timer for about 10 minutes. Close the waffle maker.
5. Check after about 5 minutes. Cook until crisp.
6. Take out the chaffle when cooked and set aside on a plate. Let it sit for a couple of minutes.
7. Repeat steps 4 – 6 and make the remaining chaffles.

# Chiffle

Serves: 4

## Ingredients:

- 2 cans chicken breast
- 1 cup shredded Mexican cheese
- 2 large eggs
- 2 tablespoons mayonnaise
- Salt to taste
- Pepper to taste

## Directions:

1. Add eggs and mayonnaise into a bowl and whisk well. Add chicken, cheese, salt and pepper and stir until well coated.
2. Preheat the mini waffle maker.
3. Spoon ¼ of the batter into the waffle maker. Set the timer for about 8 minutes. Close the waffle maker.
4. Check after about 5 minutes. Cook until crisp.
5. Take out the chaffle when cooked and set aside on a plate. Let it sit for a couple of minutes.
6. Repeat steps 3 – 5 and make the remaining chaffles.

# Savory Keto Chicken, Zucchini Chaffle

Makes: 4

## Ingredients:

- 2 ounces chicken breast, cooked, shredded
- ¼ cup shredded mozzarella
- 1 cup blanched almond flour
- ½ teaspoons baking powder
- ¼ teaspoon onion powder
- 2 tablespoons chopped green onions
- 2.5 ounces shredded zucchini, squeezed of excess moisture
- ¼ cup shredded cheddar cheese
- 1 large egg, beaten
- ½ teaspoon garlic salt
- Avocado oil cooking spray

## Directions:

1. Add chicken, zucchini, baking powder, onion powder, garlic salt, almond flour mozzarella cheese and cheddar cheese into a bowl and stir.
2. Add egg and mix well.
3. Preheat the mini waffle maker.

4. Spray avocado oil cooking spray on the bottom of the waffle maker,
5. Spoon ¼ of the batter into the waffle maker. Set the timer for about 3 - 5 minutes. Close the waffle maker.
6. Check after about 3 minutes. Cook for longer if required.
7. Take out the chaffle when cooked and set aside on a plate. Let it sit for a couple of minutes.
8. Repeat steps 5 – 7 and make the remaining chaffles.

# Chapter 3: Keto Chaffle Cake Recipes

## Chocolate Chaffle Cake

Makes: 2 cakes

**Ingredients:**

For chocolate chaffle cake:

- 4 tablespoons cocoa powder
- 2 eggs
- 2 tablespoons almond flour
- 1 teaspoon vanilla extract
- 4 tablespoons granulated swerve sweetener
- 2 tablespoons heavy whipping cream
- ½ teaspoon baking powder

For cream cheese frosting:

- 4 tablespoons cream cheese
- ¼ teaspoon vanilla extract
- 4 teaspoons swerve confectioners'
- 2 teaspoons heavy cream

**Directions:**

1. For chocolate chaffle cake: Add cocoa powder, almond flour, swerve and baking powder into a bowl and stir.
2. Stir in vanilla and heavy whipping cream
3. Beat in the eggs. Mix until well incorporated. Let the batter rest for about 5 minutes.
4. Preheat the mini waffle maker.
5. Spoon ¼ of the batter into the waffle maker. Set the timer for 4 minutes. Close the lid and cook the chaffle.
6. Remove the chaffle and place on a plate.
7. Repeat steps 6 – 7 and make the remaining chaffles.
8. Meanwhile make the cream cheese frosting as follows: Add cream cheese into a microwave safe bowl. Cook on high for about 10 seconds or until soft.
9. Add heavy whipping cream and vanilla extract into the bowl of cream cheese. Beat with an electric hand mixer until well incorporated.
10. Add confectioners swerve and continue beating until creamy and light.
11. To assemble. Place 2 chaffles on a large serving plate. Spread some frosting over it using a knife. You can also spoon the frosting into a piping bag and pipe the frosting over the chaffle.
12. Layer with one more chaffle on each. Pipe the remaining frosting over the 2nd chaffle and serve.

# Cream Cheese Carrot Cake Chaffles

Makes: 2 cakes

**Ingredients:**

- 2 eggs
- 2 tablespoons almond flour
- 1 teaspoon vanilla extract
- 2 tablespoons granulated swerve sweetener
- 1 teaspoon baking powder
- 4 tablespoons cream cheese
- 2 tablespoons finely shredded carrot
- 2 teaspoons pumpkin pie spice
- 5 – 6 tablespoons butter
- 1 tablespoon chopped walnut (optional)
- 2 tablespoons shredded coconut (optional)

For cream cheese frosting:

- 2 tablespoons cream cheese
- 2 teaspoons sugar-free syrup of your choice
- 6 tablespoons butter

**Directions:**

1. For carrot chaffle cake:

2. Add cream cheese and butter into a microwave safe bowl cook on high for 15 seconds. Whisk well.

3. Add almond flour, swerve, pumpkin pie spice and baking powder into a bowl and stir.

4. Add eggs. Beat with an electric hand mixer well incorporated. Beat in the cream cheese mixture and vanilla extract.

5. Add carrot, walnut and shredded coconut and stir.

6. Let the batter rest for about 5 minutes.

7. Preheat the mini waffle maker.

8. Spoon ¼ of the batter into the waffle maker. Set the timer for 4 minutes. Close the lid and cook the chaffle.

9. Remove the chaffle and place on a plate.

10. Repeat steps 8 – 9 and make the remaining chaffles. Let the chaffles cool completely.

11. Meanwhile make the cream cheese frosting as follows: Add cream cheese and butter into a microwave safe bowl. Cook on high for about 10 seconds or until soft. Whisk well.

12. Add sugar-free syrup into the bowl of cream cheese. Beat with an electric hand mixer until well incorporated.

13. To assemble. Place 2 chaffles on a large serving plate. Spread some frosting over it using a knife. You can also

spoon the frosting into a piping bag and pipe the frosting over the chaffle.

14. Layer with one more chaffle on each. Pipe the remaining frosting over the 2nd chaffle and serve.

# Keto Birthday Cake Chaffle

Makes: 2 cakes

**Ingredients:**

<u>For chaffle cakes:</u>

- 1 egg
- ½ teaspoon coconut flour
- 2 tablespoons almond flour
- 1 teaspoon vanilla extract
- ½ teaspoon cake batter extract
- 1 tablespoon granulated swerve sweetener
- 1 tablespoon cream cheese
- ¼ teaspoon baking powder
- 1/8 teaspoon xanthan gum
- 1 tablespoon melted butter

<u>For whipped cream vanilla frosting:</u>

- ¼ teaspoon vanilla extract
- 3 teaspoons swerve confectioners
- ¼ cup heavy cream

**Directions:**

1. To make chaffle cake: Add cream cheese and butter into a microwave safe bowl cook on high for 15 seconds. Whisk well.

2. Add almond flour, swerve, coconut flour and baking powder into a bowl and stir.

3. Add egg. Beat with an electric hand mixer well incorporated. Beat in the cream cheese mixture. Add vanilla extract, cake batter extract and xanthan gum and mix well. Let the batter rest for 1 minute.

4. Preheat the mini waffle maker.

5. Spoon ¼ of the batter into the waffle maker. Set the timer for 2 – 3 minutes. Close the lid and cook the chaffle.

6. Remove the chaffle and place on a plate.

7. Repeat steps 5 – 6 and make the remaining chaffles. Cool the chaffles completely.

8. Meanwhile make the whipped cream vanilla cheese frosting as follows: Add heavy cream, vanilla and swerve into a bowl. Beat with an electric hand mixer until soft peaks are formed.

9. To assemble: Place 2 chaffles on a large serving plate. Spread some frosting over it using a knife. You can also spoon the frosting into a piping bag and pipe the frosting over the chaffle.

10. Layer with one more chaffle on each. Pipe the remaining frosting over the 2<sup>nd</sup> chaffle and serve.

# Banana Pudding Chaffle Cake

Makes: 6 cakes

## Ingredients:

<u>For pudding:</u>

- 2 large egg yolks
- 6 tablespoons powdered swerve or erythritol
- 1 teaspoon banana extract
- 1 cup heavy whipping cream
- ½ - 1 teaspoon xanthan gum
- 1/8 teaspoon salt

<u>For banana chaffle cake:</u>

- 2 ounces cream cheese, softened
- 2 eggs, beaten
- 4 tablespoons granulated swerve sweetener
- 8 tablespoons almond flour
- ½ cup shredded mozzarella cheese
- ½ teaspoon baking powder
- 2 teaspoons banana extract

## Directions:

1. To make pudding: Add heavy cream, yolks and sweetener into a saucepan.
2. Place the saucepan over medium low. Stir constantly until the mixture is thick.
3. Add xanthan gum and mix well. Turn off the heat.
4. Stir in salt and banana extract.
5. Pour into a glass dish. Place a piece of plastic wrap directly on top of the pudding. Chill until use.
6. To make chaffle cake: Add almond flour, swerve and baking powder into a bowl and stir.
7. Add eggs. Beat with an electric hand mixer well incorporated. Beat in the cream cheese add banana extract and mix well. Let the batter rest for 5 minutes.
8. Preheat the mini waffle maker.
9. Spoon 1/6 of the batter into the waffle maker. Set the timer for 2 – 3 minutes. Close the lid and cook the chaffle.
10. Remove the chaffle and place on a plate.
11. Repeat steps 9 – 10 and make the remaining chaffles. Cool the chaffles completely.
12. Place the chaffles on individual serving plates. Top with pudding and serve.

# Pumpkin Chaffle Cake with Cream Cheese Frosting

Makes: 4 cakes

## Ingredients:

### For chaffles:

- 1 cup finely shredded mozzarella cheese
- 2 eggs
- 1 teaspoon pumpkin pie spice
- 2 tablespoons pumpkin puree

### For cream cheese frosting:

- 4 tablespoons cream cheese, softened
- 1 teaspoon clear vanilla extract
- 4 tablespoons monk fruit confectioners

## Directions:

1. Preheat the mini waffle maker.
2. Beat eggs with a fork. Add pumpkin puree and whisk well.
3. Add pumpkin pie spice into a bowl and stir until well combined. Add into the bowl of egg mixture. Whisk well.
4. Stir in mozzarella cheese.
5. Spoon about ¼ of the batter into the waffle maker. Set the timer for about 3 – 4 minutes. Close the waffle maker.

6. Take out the chaffle when cooked and set aside on a plate.

7. Repeat steps 5 – 6 and make the remaining chaffles.

8. To make cream cheese frosting: Add cream cheese, vanilla and sweetener into a bowl and whisk well.

9. To assemble: Place chaffles on a large serving plate. Spread some frosting over it using a knife. You can also spoon the frosting into a piping bag and pipe the frosting over the chaffles.

# Italian Cream Chaffle Cake

Makes: 4 cakes

## Ingredients:

<u>For chaffles:</u>

- 2 ounces cream cheese, softened
- ½ tablespoon butter, melted
- ¼ teaspoon ground cinnamon
- ½ tablespoon almond flour
- 2 tablespoons coconut flour
- ½ tablespoon shredded, unsweetened coconut
- 2 eggs
- ½ teaspoon vanilla extract
- ½ tablespoon monk fruit sweetener or any other keto friendly sweetener of your choice
- ¾ teaspoon baking powder
- ½ tablespoon chopped walnuts

<u>For Italian cream frosting:</u>

- 1 ounce cream cheese, softened
- 1 tablespoon monk fruit sweetener or any other keto friendly sweetener of your choice
- 1 tablespoon butter

- ¼ teaspoon vanilla

**Directions:**

1. Preheat the mini waffle maker.
2. Cool the melted butter to room temperature.
3. Beat eggs with a fork. Add melted butter and whisk well. Add vanilla and monk fruit sweetener and whisk well.
4. Add almond flour, baking powder, cinnamon and coconut flour into a bowl and stir until well combined. Add into the bowl of eggs. Stir until well combined.
5. Add walnuts and shredded coconut and stir.
6. Pour ¼ of the batter into the waffle maker. Set the timer for 3 – 4 minutes. Close the waffle maker.
7. Check after about 4 minutes. Cook further if required.
8. Take out the chaffle and set aside on a plate.
9. Repeat steps 6 – 8 and make the remaining chaffles. Let the chaffles cool completely.
10. To make frosting: Add cream cheese, sweetener, butter and vanilla into a bowl and whisk well.
11. Place the chaffles on a serving platter. Spread the frosting over the chaffles and serve.

# Tiramisu Chaffle Cake

Makes: 2 cakes

**Ingredients:**

<u>For chaffles:</u>

- 1 tablespoon butter, melted
- ½ ounce cream cheese, softened
- ¼ teaspoon hazelnut extract (optional)
- ½ teaspoon vanilla extract
- 2 tablespoons fine, blanched almond flour
- 1 tablespoon coconut flour
- 1 teaspoon instant coffee or espresso powder
- 1 tablespoon cacao powder
- A pinch Himalayan pink salt
- 1 large egg
- 1 tablespoon lakanto sweetener or any other keto friendly sweetener of your choice
- ½ teaspoon baking powder

<u>For frosting:</u>

- 2 ounces mascarpone cheese
- ¼ teaspoon vanilla extract
- ¼ teaspoon instant coffee

- 2 tablespoons lakanto sweetener or any other keto friendly sweetener of your choice
- 1 teaspoon cacao powder

**Directions:**

1. Preheat the mini waffle maker.
2. Cool the melted butter to room temperature.
3. Beat eggs with a fork. Add melted butter and whisk well. Add vanilla, hazelnut extract and sweetener and whisk well.
4. Add almond flour, baking powder, coconut flour, instant coffee and salt into a bowl and stir until well combined. Add into the bowl of eggs. Stir until well combined.
5. Pour ½ the batter into the waffle maker. Set the timer for 3 – 4 minutes. Close the waffle maker.
6. Check after about 4 minutes. Cook further if required.
7. Take out the chaffle and set aside on a plate.
8. Repeat steps 5 – 7 and make the remaining chaffles. Let the chaffles cool completely.
12. To make frosting: Add mascarpone cheese, lakanto, and vanilla into a bowl and whisk well. Divide the mixture into 2 bowls.
13. Add cacao and instant coffee into one of the bowls. Mix well. Leave the cream in the other bowl as it is.

14. Place the chaffles on a serving platter. Spread the frosting over the chaffles and serve.

15. Place 2 chaffles on a serving platter. Spread the cacao frosting over the chaffles.

16. Layer with a chaffle on each. Spread the plain frosting over the chaffles.

17. Chill until use.

18. Slice and serve.

## Chocolate Chip Cookie Chaffle Cake

Makes: 2 cakes

**Ingredients:**

For chocolate chip chaffle cakes:

- 2 tablespoons melted butter
- 2 egg yolks
- 2 tablespoons golden monk fruit sweetener
- ½ teaspoon cake batter extract
- ¼ teaspoon vanilla extract
- 6 tablespoons almond flour

- 2 tablespoons sugar-free chocolate chips
- ¼ teaspoon baking powder

For whipped cream frosting:

- 2 teaspoons unflavored gelatin
- 6 teaspoons swerve confectioners
- 2 cups heavy cream
- 8 teaspoons cold water

## Directions:

1. To make chocolate chip chaffle cake: Add almond flour, sweetener and baking powder into a bowl and stir.
2. Add yolks and butter and mix until well combined. Add vanilla extract, cake batter extract and chocolate chips and mix well. Let the batter rest for 1 minute.
3. Preheat the mini waffle maker.
4. Spoon ¼ of the batter into the waffle maker. Set the timer for 4 minutes. Close the lid and cook the chaffle.
5. Remove the chaffle and place on a plate.
6. Repeat steps 4 – 5 and make the remaining chaffles. Cool the chaffles completely.
7. Meanwhile make the whipped cream frosting as follows: Chill the mixing bowl and beaters in the freezer for 15 minutes.

8. Meanwhile, add cold water into a microwave safe bowl. Sprinkle gelatin on top.

9. Microwave on high for 10 seconds.

10. Remove from the microwave and whisk well.

11. Add heavy cream into the chilled bowl. Beat with an electric hand mixer on low speed until foamy. Add sweetener and beat on medium speed until soft peaks are formed.

12. Change the speed to low speed and pour the gelatin and beat until well combined.

13. Increase the speed to medium speed and beat until stiff peaks are formed. Transfer into a piping bag.

14. To assemble: Place 2 chaffles on a large serving plate. Pipe some of the frosting over the chaffle.

15. Layer with one more chaffle on each. Pipe some of the frosting over the 2nd chaffle and serve. If you have leftover frosting. Transfer into an airtight container and refrigerate until use. It can last for 4 – 5 days.

# Red Velvet Waffle Cake

Makes: 4 cakes

## Ingredients:

<u>For chaffle cakes:</u>

- 4 tablespoons Dutch processed cocoa
- 2 eggs
- ½ teaspoon baking powder
- 4 tablespoons monk fruit confectioners
- 4 drops red food coloring (optional)
- 2 tablespoons heavy whipping cream

<u>For cream cheese frosting:</u>

- 4 tablespoons cream cheese, softened
- 4 tablespoons monk fruit confectioners
- ½ teaspoon clear vanilla extract

## Directions:

1. Add eggs into a bowl and whisk well. Add cocoa, baking powder, sweetener, heavy whipping cream and red food coloring if using and whisk until well combined.
2. Let the batter rest for 1 minute.
3. Preheat the mini waffle maker.

4. Spoon ¼ of the batter into the waffle maker. Set the timer for 4 minutes. Close the lid and cook the chaffle.
5. Remove the chaffle and place on a plate.
6. Repeat steps 4 – 5 and make the remaining chaffles. Cool the chaffles completely.
7. To make cream cheese frosting: Add cream cheese, vanilla and sweetener into a bowl and whisk well.
8. To assemble: Place chaffles on a large serving plate. Spread some frosting over it using a knife. You can also spoon the frosting into a piping bag and pipe the frosting over the chaffles.
9. Cut into slices and serve.

# Boston Cream Pie Chaffle Cake

Makes: 2 cakes

## Ingredients:

<u>For chaffle cakes:</u>

- 1 tablespoon cream cheese, softened
- ¼ teaspoon vanilla extract
- 10 drops Boston cream extract
- 1 egg
- ½ teaspoon coconut flour
- 2 tablespoons almond flour
- 1 tablespoon butter, melted
- 1 tablespoon swerve sweetener or any other keto friendly sweetener of your choice
- ¼ teaspoon baking powder
- 1/8 teaspoon xanthan powder

<u>For pudding:</u>

- 1 egg yolk
- ¾ tablespoon powdered swerve or erythritol
- ¼ teaspoon vanilla extract
- ¼ cup heavy whipping cream
- A pinch xanthan gum

For ganache:

- 1 tablespoon heavy whipping cream
- ½ tablespoon swerve confectioners
- 1 tablespoon chopped unsweetened baking chocolate bar

## Directions:

1. To make pudding: Add heavy cream, yolks and sweetener into a saucepan.
2. Place the saucepan over medium low. Stir constantly until the mixture is thick.
3. Add xanthan gum and mix well. Turn off the heat.
4. Stir in salt and banana extract.
5. Pour into a glass dish. Place a piece of plastic wrap directly on top of the pudding. Chill until use.
6. Preheat the mini waffle maker.
7. Cool the melted butter to room temperature.
8. Beat egg with a fork. Add melted butter and whisk well. Add cream cheese, vanilla, Boston cream extract and sweetener and whisk well.
9. Add almond flour, baking powder, coconut flour and salt into a bowl and stir until well combined. Add into the bowl of egg. Stir until well combined.
10. Sprinkle xanthan flour and whisk until well combined.

11. Pour ½ the batter into the waffle maker. Set the timer for 3 – 4 minutes. Close the waffle maker.

12. Check after about 4 minutes. Cook further if required.

13. Take out the chaffle and set aside on a plate.

14. Repeat steps 11 – 13 and make the remaining chaffles. Let the chaffles cool completely.

15. To make ganache: Add heavy cream, swerve and chocolate into a microwave safe bowl. Microwave on high for 20 seconds. Stir well. If the mixture is not melted, cook for another 10 – 20 seconds or until melted completely.

16. Place the chaffles on individual serving plates. Spoon some pudding over the chaffles. Drizzle ganache on top and serve.

# Keto Lemon Chaffle Cake

Makes: 2 cakes

## Ingredients:

For chaffles cake:

- 1 ounce cream cheese, softened
- ¼ teaspoon lemon extract
- 1 egg
- 1 tablespoon coconut flour
- 1 teaspoon butter, melted
- ½ teaspoon monk fruit confectioners blend
- 10 drops cake batter extract
- ½ teaspoon baking powder
- 1/8 teaspoon xanthan powder

For frosting:

- ½ tablespoon monk fruit confectioners blend
- ¼ cup heavy whipping cream
- 1/8 teaspoon lemon extract
- ¼ teaspoon grated lemon zest

## Directions:

1. Add cream cheese, lemon extract, egg, coconut flour, butter, monk fruit sweetener, cake batter extract, baking powder and xanthan gum into a mixing bowl. Beat with an electric mixer until smooth.
2. Plug in the mini waffle maker and let it preheat.
3. Pour ½ the batter into the waffle maker. Set the timer for 3 – 4 minutes. Close the waffle maker.
4. Check after about 4 minutes. Cook further if required.
5. Take out the chaffle and set aside on a plate.
6. Repeat steps 11 – 13 and make the remaining chaffles. Let the chaffles cool completely.
7. To make frosting: Chill the mixing bowl and beaters in the freezer for 15 minutes.
8. Add heavy cream into the chilled bowl. Beat with an electric hand mixer on low speed until foamy. Add sweetener and beat on medium speed until soft peaks are formed.
9. Add lemon extract and lemon zest and fold gently.
10. To assemble: Place chaffles on a large serving plate. Spread some frosting over it using a knife. You can also spoon the frosting into a piping bag and pipe the frosting over the chaffles.
11. Cut into slices and serve.

# Peanut Butter Chaffle Cake

Makes: 4 cakes

## Ingredients:

<u>For peanut butter chaffle cake:</u>

- 2 eggs
- ½ teaspoon baking powder
- 4 tablespoons monk fruit confectioners
- 2 tablespoons heavy whipping cream
- 4 tablespoons sugar-free peanut butter powder
- ½ teaspoon peanut butter extract

<u>For peanut butter frosting:</u>

- 4 tablespoons monk fruit confectioners
- 2 tablespoons sugar-free natural peanut butter or peanut butter powder
- ½ teaspoon vanilla
- 2 tablespoons butter, softened
- 4 tablespoons cream cheese, softened

## Directions:

1. Preheat the mini waffle maker.

2. Beat eggs with a fork. Add cream and sweetener and whisk well.

3. Add peanut butter powder, coconut flour and salt into a bowl and stir until well combined. Add into the bowl of egg. Stir until well combined.

4. Add peanut butter extract and peanut butter powder and whisk well. Let the batter rest for a couple of minutes.

5. Pour ½ the batter into the waffle maker. Set the timer for 3 – 4 minutes. Close the waffle maker.

6. Check after about 4 minutes. Cook further if required.

7. Take out the chaffle and set aside on a plate.

8. Repeat steps 5 – 7 and make the remaining chaffles. Let the chaffles cool completely.

9. To make peanut butter frosting: Add cream cheese, butter, vanilla, peanut butter and sweetener into a bowl and whisk well with an electric hand mixer until well combined.

10. To assemble: Place chaffles on a large serving plate. Spread some frosting over it using a knife. You can also spoon the frosting into a piping bag and pipe the frosting over the chaffles.

11. Cut into slices and serve.

# Cap'n Crunch Cereal Chaffle Cake

Makes: 4 cakes

<u>For chaffle cakes:</u>

- 2 eggs
- 1 teaspoon coconut flour
- 4 tablespoons almond flour
- 2 tablespoons butter, melted
- 40 drops Captain cereal flavoring
- 2 tablespoon swerve confectioners
- ½ teaspoon baking powder
- ¼ teaspoon xanthan powder
- 1 tablespoon cream cheese, softened
- ½ teaspoon vanilla extract

<u>To serve:</u>

- Melted butter
- Sugar-free syrup

## Directions:

1. Add cream cheese, eggs, coconut flour, almond flour, butter, vanilla, Captain Cereal flavoring, baking powder

and xanthan gum into a mixing bowl. Beat with an electric mixer until smooth.

2. Plug in the mini waffle maker and let it preheat.

3. Pour ¼ of the batter into the waffle maker. Set the timer for 3 – 4 minutes. Close the waffle maker.

4. Check after about 4 minutes. Cook further if required.

5. Take out the chaffle and set aside on a plate.

6. Repeat steps 3 – 5 and make the remaining chaffles. Let the chaffles cool completely.

7. Brush with some butter and serve with some sugar-free syrup of your choice.

# Chapter 4: Keto Savory Chaffles

## Spicy Jalapeno Popper Chaffles

Makes: 4 chaffles

### Ingredients:

- 1 cup finely shredded cheddar cheese
- 2 large eggs
- 2 ounces cream cheese
- 1 tablespoon chopped jalapeños
- 4 tablespoons bacon bits
- ½ teaspoon baking powder (optional)

### Directions:

1. Add cream cheese into a microwave safe bowl cook on high for 15 seconds.
2. Add egg. Beat with an electric hand mixer well incorporated.
3. Add baking powder and whisk well. Add jalapeños and bacon bits and stir. Let the batter rest for 1 minute.
4. Preheat the mini waffle maker.

5. Spoon ¼ of the batter into the waffle maker. Set the timer for 3 – 4 minutes. Close the lid and cook the chaffle. Cook for longer if you want crisp chaffles.
6. Remove the chaffle and place on a plate.
7. Repeat steps 5 – 6 and make the remaining chaffles.
8. Serve with some toppings if desired.

## Garlic Parmesan Chaffles

Makes: 4

**Ingredients:**

- 1 cup shredded mozzarella cheese
- 2 large eggs
- 1 teaspoon Italian seasoning
- 2/3 cup grated Parmesan cheese
- 2 cloves garlic, minced
- ½ teaspoon baking powder (optional)

**Directions:**

1. Preheat the mini waffle maker.
2. Beat eggs with a fork. Stir in the mozzarella, Italian seasoning, Parmesan cheese, garlic and baking powder.

3. Spoon ¼ of the batter into the waffle maker. Set the timer for 2 to 3 minutes. Close the waffle maker.

4. Take out the chaffle and set aside on a plate. Let it sit for a couple of minutes.

5. Repeat steps 3 – 4 and make the remaining chaffles.

# Keto Cornbread Chaffle

Makes: 4

**Ingredients:**

- 1 cup shredded mozzarella cheese or cheddar cheese
- 2 large eggs
- 10 – 12 slices jalapeños
- 1/8 teaspoon salt
- ½ teaspoon corn extract
- 2 teaspoons Frank's red hot sauce

**Directions:**

1. Preheat the mini waffle maker.
2. Beat eggs with a fork. Stir in the mozzarella, jalapeños, salt, corn extract and hot sauce.
3. Spoon ¼ of the batter into the waffle maker. Set the timer for 2 to 3 minutes. Close the waffle maker.
4. Take out the chaffle and set aside on a plate. Let it sit for a couple of minutes.
5. Repeat steps 3 – 4 and make the remaining chaffles.

# Keto Taco Chaffle

Makes: 4 chaffles

## Ingredients:

- 1 cup shredded mozzarella cheese or cheddar cheese
- ½ teaspoon Italian seasoning
- 2 large eggs

For taco filling:

- 2 pounds ground beef or turkey
- 2 teaspoons chili powder
- 1 teaspoon garlic powder
- ½ teaspoon onion powder
- 3 teaspoons smoked paprika
- 2 teaspoons ground cumin
- 1 teaspoon cocoa powder
- ½ teaspoon salt or to taste

For toppings:

- Lettuce
- Cheese
- Tomatoes
- Any other toppings of your choice

## Directions:

1. Place a skillet over medium heat. Add beef and cook until brown. Add rest of the ingredients for filling and mix well. Turn off the heat.
2. To make chaffles: Preheat the mini waffle maker.
3. Beat eggs with a fork. Stir in the mozzarella and Italian seasoning.
4. Spoon ¼ of the batter into the waffle maker. Set the timer for 2 to 3 minutes. Close the waffle maker.
5. Take out the chaffle and set aside on a plate. Let it sit for a couple of minutes.
6. Repeat steps 4 – 5 and make the remaining chaffles.
7. Top with taco meat and serve with suggested toppings.

# Chaffle Garlic Cheesy Breadsticks

Makes: 16 breadsticks

## Ingredients:

- 1 cup shredded mozzarella cheese
- 2 eggs
- 4 tablespoons almond flour
- Salt to taste
- 2/3 cup grated Parmesan cheese
- 2 large cloves garlic, minced or 1 teaspoon garlic powder

For topping:

- 4 tablespoons unsalted butter, softened
- ½ cup grated mozzarella cheese
- 1 teaspoon garlic powder

## Directions:

1. Preheat the mini waffle maker.
2. Beat eggs with a fork. Stir in the mozzarella, garlic, almond flour, Parmesan cheese and salt.
3. Spoon ¼ of the batter into the waffle maker. Set the timer for 5 minutes. Close the waffle maker.

4. Take out the chaffle and set aside on your cutting board. Cut into 4 strips.

5. Repeat steps 3 – 4 and make the remaining chaffles.

6. Place the sticks on a baking sheet.

7. Add butter and garlic powder into a bowl and stir. Spread this mixture over the sticks.

8. Sprinkle cheese on top of the sticks

9. Set the oven to broil mode and preheat the oven. Broil for a couple of minutes until the cheese melts.

10. Serve right away.

# Chaffle Bruschetta

Makes: 4 chaffles

## Ingredients:

- 1 cup shredded mozzarella cheese
- 2 large eggs
- 1 teaspoon Italian seasoning
- 2/3 cup grated Parmesan cheese
- 2 cloves garlic, minced
- ½ teaspoon baking powder (optional)

For topping:

- 8 cherry tomatoes, chopped
- Olive oil to drizzle
- 1/8 teaspoon salt
- 1 teaspoon finely chopped basil

## Directions:

1. Preheat the mini waffle maker.
2. Beat eggs with a fork. Stir in the mozzarella, Italian seasoning, Parmesan cheese, garlic and baking powder.
3. Spoon ¼ of the batter into the waffle maker. Set the timer for 2 to 3 minutes. Close the waffle maker.

4. Take out the chaffle and set aside on a plate. Let it sit for a couple of minutes.
5. Repeat steps 3 – 4 and make the remaining chaffles.
6. Place chaffles on a serving platter.
7. To make bruschetta topping: Add tomatoes, salt and basil into a bowl. Toss well.
8. Drizzle oil on top. Toss well.
9. Top over the chaffles and serve.

# Sweet and Spicy Chaffle

Makes: 4 chaffles

## Ingredients:

- 1 cup shredded mozzarella cheese or cheddar cheese
- 2 large eggs
- 1/8 teaspoon salt or to taste
- ¼ teaspoon cayenne pepper
- 4 tablespoons lakanto maple syrup
- 1 teaspoon smoked paprika

## Directions:

1. Preheat the mini waffle maker.
2. Beat eggs with a fork. Stir in the mozzarella, salt, paprika and cayenne pepper.
3. Spoon ¼ of the batter into the waffle maker. Set the timer for 2 to 3 minutes. Close the waffle maker.
4. Take out the chaffle and set aside on a plate. Let it sit for a couple of minutes.
5. Repeat steps 3 – 4 and make the remaining chaffles.
6. Drizzle lakanto maple syrup on top and serve.

# Savory Herb Chaffle

Makes: 4 chaffles

## Ingredients:

- ½ cup shredded mozzarella cheese
- 2 large eggs
- 2 teaspoons herb seasoning
- ½ cup grated Parmesan cheese
- 2 cloves garlic, minced
- ¼ teaspoon salt or to taste

## Directions:

1. Preheat the mini waffle maker.
2. Beat eggs with a fork. Stir in the mozzarella, herb seasoning, Parmesan cheese, garlic and salt.
3. Spoon ¼ of the batter into the waffle maker. Set the timer for 2 to 3 minutes. Close the waffle maker.
4. Take out the chaffle when cooked and set aside on a plate. Let it sit for a couple of minutes.
5. Repeat steps 3 – 4 and make the remaining chaffles.

# Jicama Hash Brown Chaffle

Makes: 2 chaffles

## Ingredients:

- 1 medium jicama, peeled, shredded
- 1 garlic clove, pressed
- 1 egg
- 1 small onion minced
- ½ cup shredded cheese of your choice
- Salt to taste
- Pepper to taste

Toppings:

- Sour cream
- Bacon bits
- Chopped chives
- Shredded cheese

## Directions:

1. Sprinkle salt over the jicama. Toss well and place in a colander. Let it sit for 15 minutes.
2. Squeeze the jicama of excess moisture.

3. Place in a microwave safe bowl. Cook on high for about 5 minutes or until tender.

4. To make chaffles: Beat egg with a fork. Add garlic, onion, cheese, salt and pepper and mix well.

5. Preheat the waffle maker.

6. Scatter some mozzarella cheese on the waffle maker.

6. Pour ½ the batter. Set the timer for 7 minutes. Close the waffle maker. Flip sides after 5 minutes.

7. Take out the chaffle when cooked and set aside on a plate. Let it sit for a couple of minutes.

8. Repeat steps 5 – 7 and make the other chaffle.

9. Serve with suggested toppings.

# Chaffle Breadsticks

## Ingredients:

- 1 cup shredded mozzarella cheese
- ½ cup grated Parmesan cheese
- 2 large eggs
- ½ teaspoon garlic powder

To serve:

- Olive oil, to drizzle
- Grated Parmesan cheese
- Minced fresh herbs

## Directions:

1. Preheat the mini waffle maker.
2. Beat eggs with a fork. Stir in the mozzarella, Italian seasoning, Parmesan cheese and garlic powder.
3. Spoon ¼ of the batter into the waffle maker. Set the timer for 2 to 3 minutes. Close the waffle maker.
4. Take out the chaffle and set aside on a plate. Let it sit for a couple of minutes.
5. Repeat steps 3 – 4 and make the remaining chaffles.
6. Cut the chaffles into strips.

7. Place on a baking sheet. Bake for a few minutes in the oven.

8. Place the bread sticks on a serving platter. Drizzle olive oil on top. Sprinkle Parmesan cheese and fresh herbs and serve.

# Fried Pickle Chaffle Sticks

Makes: 4 chaffles

## Ingredients:

- 1 cup shredded mozzarella cheese
- 2 large eggs
- 2 tablespoons pickle juice
- ½ cup pork panko
- 12 – 15 thin pickle slices, pat dried with paper towels

## Directions:

1. Preheat the mini waffle maker.
2. Beat eggs with a fork. Stir in the mozzarella, pickle juice and pork panko.
3. Spoon ¼ of the batter into the waffle maker. Scatter 3 – 4 pickle slices. Set the timer for 4 minutes. Close the waffle maker.
4. Take out the chaffle when cooked and set aside on a plate.
5. Repeat steps 3 – 4 and make the remaining chaffles.
6. Cut each into 4 sticks and serve.

# Italian Chaffle Sandwich

Makes: 2 sandwiches

## Ingredients:

- 1 cup shredded mozzarella cheese
- ½ cup grated Parmesan cheese
- 2 large eggs
- ½ teaspoon garlic powder
- 2 teaspoons Italian seasoning
- 1 roasted red pepper, chopped
- 2 tablespoons chopped ham
- Lettuce leaves

## Directions:

1. Preheat the mini waffle maker.
2. Beat eggs with a fork. Stir in the mozzarella, Italian seasoning, Parmesan cheese and garlic powder.
3. Spoon ¼ of the batter into the waffle maker. Set the timer for 2 to 3 minutes. Close the waffle maker.
4. Take out the chaffle and set aside on a plate. Let it sit for a couple of minutes.
5. Repeat steps 3 – 4 and make the remaining chaffles.

6. Place 2 chaffles on a serving platter. Top with lettuce leaves, ham and red pepper. Cover with the remaining chaffles and serve.

# BLT Chaffle Sandwich

Makes: 2 sandwiches

## Ingredients:

<u>For chaffle:</u>

- 1 cup shredded mozzarella cheese
- 2 tablespoons sliced green onion
- 2 large eggs
- 1 teaspoon Italian seasoning
- Salt to taste

<u>For filling:</u>

- Cooked bacon
- 2 tablespoons mayonnaise
- Few lettuce leaves
- 1 tomato, thinly sliced

## Directions:

1. Preheat the mini waffle maker.
2. Beat eggs and Italian seasoning with a fork. Stir in the mozzarella, green and green onion.
3. Sprinkle some extra mozzarella cheese on the bottom of the waffle maker.

4. Spoon ¼ of the batter into the waffle maker. Sprinkle some more cheese on top. Set the timer for 4 minutes. Close the waffle maker.
5. Take out the chaffle when cooked and set aside on a plate.
6. Repeat steps 4 – 5 and make the remaining chaffles.
7. Place 2 chaffles on a serving plate. Spread a tablespoon of mayonnaise on each.
8. Place bacon, lettuce leaves and tomato slices over it. Cover with the remaining 2 chaffles and serve.

# Chaffle Breakfast Sandwich

Makes: 2 sandwiches

## Ingredients:

- 2 eggs
- 2 tablespoons almond flour
- 1 cup Monterey Jack cheese
- 4 tablespoons butter

## Directions:

1. Preheat the mini waffle maker.
2. Add eggs into a bowl and whisk with a fork. Add almond flour and cheese and whisk well.
3. Spoon ¼ of the batter into the waffle maker. Set the timer for 3 to 4 minutes. Close the waffle maker.
4. Take out the chaffle and set aside on a plate.
5. Repeat steps 2 – 3 and make the remaining chaffles.
6. Place a skillet over medium heat. Add 2 tablespoons butter. When butter melts, place 2 chaffles and until crisp. Press lightly while cooking. Flip sides and cook the other side until crisp.
7. Remove onto a plate. Let it rest for a couple of minutes before serving.

# Avocado Toast

Makes: 2 chaffles

## Ingredients:

For chaffle:

- 1 cup finely shredded mozzarella cheese
- 2 large eggs
- 2 teaspoons baking powder
- 2 tablespoons almond flour

For avocado topping:

- 1 avocado, peeled, pitted, chopped
- 2 teaspoons lemon juice
- Pepper to taste
- Salt to taste
- 2 teaspoons butter, melted
- ½ cup feta cheese

## Directions:

1. Preheat the regular waffle maker.
2. Beat eggs with a fork.

3. Add almond flour and baking powder into a bowl and stir until well combined. Add into the bowl of eggs. Stir until well combined.

4. Stir in mozzarella cheese.

5. Spoon ½ the batter into the waffle maker. Set the timer for about 2 – 3 minutes. Close the waffle maker.

6. Check after about 5 minutes. Cook for longer if required.

7. Take out the chaffle when cooked and set aside on a plate. Let it sit for a couple of minutes.

8. Repeat steps 5 – 6 and make the other chaffle.

9. Place chaffles on a plate and brush with melted butter.

10. Meanwhile, add avocado, lemon juice, salt, pepper and feta cheese into a bowl and toss well.

11. Divide the avocado mixture among the chaffles. Spread it on one half of the chaffle. Fold the other half over the filling and serve.

## Zucchini Chaffles

Makes: 4 chaffles

**Ingredients:**

For chaffle:

- 2 cups shredded zucchini
- ½ cup shredded mozzarella cheese
- 1 cup shredded Parmesan cheese or more if required
- 2 eggs
- 2 teaspoons dried basil or 2 tablespoons chopped, fresh basil
- Salt to taste
- Pepper to taste

## Directions:

1. Place zucchini in a colander. Sprinkle salt over it. Mix well with your hands. Set aside for 15 minutes.
2. Squeeze the zucchini of excess moisture.
3. Plug on the mini waffle maker and allow it to preheat.
4. Beat eggs in a bowl.
5. Add zucchini, mozzarella cheese, salt, pepper and basil to the bowl of eggs and whisk well.
6. Preheat the waffle maker.
7. Scatter ¼ of the Parmesan cheese on bottom of the waffle maker initially.
8. Close the lid and let it cook for half a minute.
9. Next pour ¼ of the egg mixture. Sprinkle some more cheese over the egg mixture if desired.

10. Set the timer for 4 – 6 minutes. Check after about 4 to 5 minutes. Cook for a few more minutes if it looks uncooked.
11. Remove onto a plate and let it cool for a couple of minutes.
12. Repeat steps 7 – 11 and make the remaining chaffles.

# Cauliflower Chaffles

Makes: 4 chaffles

## Ingredients:

- 2 cups grated cauliflower (grated to rice like texture)
- 1 cup shredded mozzarella cheese or Mexican cheese blend
- 2 large eggs
- 1 teaspoon Italian seasoning
- 1 cup grated Parmesan cheese or more if required
- 2 cloves garlic, minced or ½ teaspoon garlic powder
- ½ teaspoon salt or to taste
- ½ teaspoon pepper or to taste
- ½ teaspoon baking powder (optional)

## Directions:

1. Preheat the mini waffle maker.
2. Add all the ingredients except Parmesan cheese into a blender and blend until fairly smooth. Pour into a bowl.
3. Sprinkle 2 tablespoons Parmesan cheese on the bottom of the waffle maker.
4. Spoon ¼ of the batter into the waffle maker. Set the timer for 4 to 6 minutes. Close the waffle maker.

5. Take out the chaffle and set aside on a plate. Let it sit for a couple of minutes.
6. Repeat steps 3 – 5 and make the remaining chaffles.

# Okra Fritter Chaffle

Makes: 4 chaffles

## Ingredients:

- ½ cup shredded mozzarella cheese or more if required
- 2 eggs
- 8 tablespoons almond flour
- 4 tablespoons heavy cream
- 1 teaspoon onion powder
- 2 tablespoons keto friendly mayonnaise
- 1 tablespoon keto friendly creole seasoning
- 2 cups sliced okra, thaw if frozen
- Salt to taste
- Pepper to taste

## Directions:

1. Preheat the mini waffle maker.
2. Add eggs, cream, mayonnaise, salt, pepper and creole seasoning into a bowl and whisk well.
3. Add almond flour. Stir until well combined.
4. Stir in okra. Let the batter sit for 10 minutes.
5. Sprinkle a little mozzarella on the bottom of the waffle maker.

6. Spoon ¼ of the batter into the waffle maker. Set the timer for about 5 minutes. Close the waffle maker.
7. Check after about 5 minutes. Cook for longer if you want it crisp.
8. Take out the chaffle when cooked and set aside on a plate. Let it sit for a couple of minutes.
9. Repeat steps 5 – 8 and make the remaining chaffles.
10. Sprinkle a little salt on top and serve.

# Broccoli and Cheese Chaffle

Makes: 4 chaffles

## Ingredients:

- 1 cup shredded cheddar cheese
- 2 eggs
- 2 tablespoons almond flour
- ½ cup chopped broccoli
- ½ teaspoon garlic powder
- Salt to taste

## Directions:

1. Preheat the mini waffle maker.
2. Add eggs, salt and garlic powder into a bowl and whisk well.
3. Add almond flour. Stir until well combined.
4. Stir in broccoli. Let the batter sit for 10 minutes.
5. Spoon ¼ of the batter into the waffle maker. Set the timer for about 5 minutes. Close the waffle maker.
6. Check after about 5 minutes. Cook for longer if you want it crisp.
7. Take out the chaffle when cooked and set aside on a plate. Let it sit for a couple of minutes.
8. Repeat steps 5 – 8 and make the remaining chaffles.

9. Serve as it is or with sour cream or keto friendly ranch dressing.

# Spinach & Ricotta Chaffle

Makes: 4 chaffles

## Ingredients:

- 8 ounces frozen spinach, thawed, squeezed of excess moisture
- 1 cup shredded mozzarella cheese
- 2 large eggs
- ½ cup grated Parmesan cheese
- 2 cloves garlic or ½ teaspoon garlic powder
- Salt to taste
- Pepper to taste

## Directions:

1. Preheat the mini waffle maker.
2. Add eggs, salt, pepper and garlic powder into a bowl and whisk well.
3. Add Parmesan cheese and mozzarella cheese. Stir until well combined.
4. Stir in spinach. Let the batter sit for 10 minutes.
5. Spoon ¼ of the batter into the waffle maker. Set the timer for about 5 minutes. Close the waffle maker.

6. Check after about 5 minutes. Cook for longer if you want it crisp.
7. Take out the chaffle when cooked and set aside on a plate. Let it sit for a couple of minutes.
8. Repeat steps 5 – 8 and make the remaining chaffles.

# Bacon, Egg and Cheese Chaffle

Makes: 2

## Ingredients:

- 1 egg
- 1 slice cooked chopped bacon
- 6 tablespoons grated cheese

## Directions:

1. Preheat a regular waffle maker.
2. Beat eggs with a fork. Add bacon and cheese and whisk well.
3. Spoon ½ the batter into the waffle maker. Set the timer for about 2 – 3 minutes. Close the waffle maker.
4. Check after about 5 minutes. Cook for longer if you want it crisp.
5. Take out the chaffle when cooked and set aside on a plate. Let it sit for a couple of minutes.
6. Repeat steps 3 – 5 and make the remaining chaffles.

# Everything Bagel Chaffles

Makes: 4 chaffles

## Ingredients:

- 2 cups shredded mozzarella cheese
- 2 eggs
- 2 tablespoons almond flour
- 2 teaspoons baking powder
- Salt to taste
- 4 teaspoons everything bagel seasoning
- ½ teaspoon onion powder
- ½ teaspoon garlic powder

## Directions:

1. Preheat the mini waffle maker.
2. Add eggs, salt, everything bagel seasoning, onion powder and garlic powder into a bowl and whisk well.
3. Add almond flour. Stir until well combined.
4. Stir in mozzarella cheese. Let the batter sit for 10 minutes.
5. Spoon ¼ of the batter into the waffle maker. Set the timer for about 5 minutes. Close the waffle maker.
6. Check after about 5 minutes. Cook for longer if you want it crisp.

7. Take out the chaffle when cooked and set aside on a plate. Let it sit for a couple of minutes.
8. Repeat steps 5 – 8 and make the remaining chaffles.

# Corndog Chaffle

Makes: 6 chaffles

## Ingredients:

- 2 egg whites or 2 flax eggs (2 tablespoons ground flaxseeds mixed with 6 tablespoons water)
- 4 teaspoons granulated swerve or any other keto friendly sweetener of your choice
- ½ teaspoon baking powder
- 4 heaping tablespoons Mexican blend cheese
- 30 to 40 drops cornbread flavoring
- 3 tablespoons butter, melted
- 6 tablespoons almond flour
- 2 egg yolks
- 2 tablespoons chopped, pickled jalapeños

## Directions:

1. If you are using flax eggs, set aside the mixture for 15 minutes.
2. Preheat the mini waffle maker.
3. Add egg whites or flax eggs, swerve, baking powder, cheese, cornbread flavoring, butter and yolks into a bowl and whisk well.

4. Add almond flour. Stir until well combined.
5. Stir in jalapeños. Let the batter sit for 10 minutes.
6. Sprinkle some cheese on the bottom of the waffle maker. Spoon 1/6 of the batter into the waffle maker. Sprinkle some more cheese on top of the batter.
7. Set the timer for about 5 minutes. Close the waffle maker.
8. Check after about 5 minutes. Cook for longer if you want it crisp.
9. Take out the chaffle when cooked and set aside on a plate. Let it sit for a couple of minutes.
10. Repeat steps 6 – 9 and make the remaining chaffles.

# Sloppy Joe Chaffle

Makes: 4

## Ingredients:

<u>For chaffle:</u>

- 1 cup finely shredded mozzarella cheese
- 2 eggs
- 4 tablespoons almond flour
- ½ teaspoon baking powder
- 1 teaspoon psyllium husk powder

<u>For Sloppy Joe:</u>

- 2 pounds ground beef
- 2 teaspoons minced garlic
- 1 teaspoon salt or to taste
- 2 tablespoons chili powder
- 1 cup beef broth
- 2 teaspoons mustard powder
- 1 teaspoon paprika
- 2 teaspoons onion powder
- 6 tablespoons tomato paste
- ½ teaspoon pepper or to taste
- 2 teaspoons cocoa powder

- 2 teaspoons coconut aminos
- 2 teaspoons swerve brown
- Salt to taste

## Directions:

1. To make Sloppy Joes: Place a skillet over medium heat. Add beef, salt and pepper and cook until brown. Break it simultaneously as it cooks.

2. Add garlic, chili powder, broth, mustard powder, paprika, onion powder, tomato paste, pepper, cocoa, coconut, swerve and salt. Mix well. When it begins to boil, lower the heat and simmer for a few minutes until thick. Turn off the heat.

3. Preheat the mini waffle maker.

4. Beat eggs with a fork.

5. Add almond flour, baking powder and psyllium husk powder into a bowl and stir until well combined. Add into the bowl of eggs. Whisk well.

6. Stir in mozzarella cheese.

7. Sprinkle some cheese on the bottom of the waffle maker. Close the waffle maker and let it cook for 30 seconds.

8. Spoon ¼ of the batter into the waffle maker. Set the timer for about 6 - 8 minutes. Close the waffle maker.

9. Check after about 5 minutes. Cook until crisp.

10. Take out the chaffle and set aside on a plate. Let it sit for a couple of minutes.

11. Repeat steps 7 – 10 and make the remaining chaffles.

12. Spread Sloppy Joes on top and serve. Leftover Sloppy Joes can be stored in an airtight container in the refrigerator. It can be used in some other recipe like tacos or over lettuce leaves etc.

# Crispy Everything Bagel Chaffle Chips

Makes: 12 chips

## Ingredients:

- 2 teaspoons Everything Bagel seasoning
- 6 tablespoons shredded Parmesan cheese

## Directions:

1. Plug in the mini waffle maker and let it preheat.
2. Sprinkle 2 tablespoons of Parmesan cheese in the waffle maker. Close the lid and set the timer for 3 minutes. Uncover and check after 3 minutes. Cook for longer if it is not crisp.
3. Remove from the waffle maker and set aside on a plate. Let it rest for a few minutes to cool.
4. Repeat steps 2 – 3 and make the remaining chips.
5. Cool completely and serve.

# Chaffle Stuffing

Makes: 8

**Ingredients:**

For chaffle:

- 4 eggs
- 1 cup shredded mozzarella cheese
- ½ teaspoon salt or to taste to taste
- 1 teaspoon dried poultry seasoning
- 1 teaspoon onion powder
- ½ teaspoon garlic powder
- ½ teaspoon pepper

For stuffing:

- 2 small onions, diced
- 8 ounces mushrooms, diced
- 6 eggs, beaten
- 4 celery stalks
- 8 tablespoons butter

## Directions:

1. Preheat the mini waffle maker.
2. Add eggs, salt, pepper, poultry seasoning, onion powder and garlic powder into a bowl and whisk well.
3. Add almond flour. Stir until well combined.
4. Stir in mozzarella cheese. Let the batter sit for 10 minutes.
5. Spoon 1/8 of the batter into the waffle maker. Set the timer for about 5 minutes. Close the waffle maker.
6. Check after about 5 minutes. Cook for longer if you want it crisp.
7. Take out the chaffle when cooked and set aside on a plate.
8. Repeat steps 5 – 8 and make the remaining chaffles. Chop or tear the chaffles and add into a bowl.
9. To make stuffing: Place a nonstick pan over medium heat. Add butter. When butter melts, add onions and celery and sauté for a couple of minutes.
10. Add mushrooms and cook until tender.
11. Turn off the heat and transfer into the bowl of chaffles. Pour eggs over it and mix until well incorporated. Transfer into a casserole dish.
12. Bake in a preheated oven at 375°F for about 25-30 minutes.
13. Remove from the oven and cool for a few minutes before serving.

# Keto Sausage Ball Chaffle

Makes: 8

## Ingredients:

- 2 cups shredded Sharp cheddar cheese
- 2 large eggs
- ½ cup grated Parmesan cheese
- 2 cups almond flour
- 4 teaspoons baking powder
- 2 pounds bulk Italian sausage

To serve: Use any (optional)

- Sour cream
- Keto friendly marinara sauce
- Keto friendly ranch dressing
- Sugar-free maple syrup

## Directions:

1. Preheat the mini waffle maker.
2. Beat eggs with a fork. Add cheddar cheese, Parmesan cheese, baking powder, Italian sausage and almond flour. Mix well using your hands.

3. Spoon 3 tablespoons of the batter into the waffle maker. Set the timer for 3- 4 minutes. Close the waffle maker.

4. Flip sides and cook for 2 minutes. Take out the chaffle and set aside on a plate. Let it sit for a couple of minutes.

5. Repeat steps 3 – 4 and make the remaining chaffles.

# Bacon Cheddar Bay Biscuits Chaffle

Makes: 10 – 12

## Ingredients:

- ½ cup oat fiber
- 1 cup almond flour
- 2 eggs, beaten
- 6 strips bacon, cooked, crumbled
- ½ cup sour cream
- 3 tablespoons butter, melted
- 1 cup smoked gouda cheese, shredded
- 1 cup shredded sharp cheddar cheese
- 1 teaspoon garlic salt
- 1 tablespoon dried parsley
- 1 teaspoon onion powder
- ½ teaspoon baking soda
- 1 tablespoon baking powder
- 2 tablespoons bacon grease, melted
- ½ teaspoon swerve confectioners

## Directions:

1. Preheat the mini waffle maker.

2. Add eggs, sour cream, bacon grease, butter, parsley, bacon and both the cheeses into a bowl and whisk well.

3. Add almond flour, oat fiber, baking powder, baking soda, swerve, garlic salt and onion powder into a bowl and stir until well combined. Add into the bowl of egg mixture. Whisk well.

4. Transfer into the bowl of wet ingredients and whisk until well combined.

5. Spoon about 3 tablespoons of the batter into the waffle maker. Set the timer for about 5 to 6 minutes. Close the waffle maker.

6. Check after about 5 minutes. Cook longer if necessary.

7. Take out the chaffle and set aside on a plate.

8. Repeat steps 5 – 7 and make the remaining chaffles.

# Savory Chaffles with Ham and Jalapenos

Makes: 2 chaffles

## Ingredients:

- 1 ounce sharp cheddar cheese, finely grated
- 1 large egg
- ½ scallion, finely chopped
- 1 jalapeño pepper or use lesser if you do not like hot, deseeded, finely grated
- 1 ounce ham steak, finely chopped
- 1 teaspoon coconut flour

## Directions:

1. Add egg into a bowl and whisk well. Add cheese, scallion, jalapeño and ham steak.
2. Preheat the mini waffle maker.
3. Spoon ¼ of the batter into the waffle maker. Set the timer for about 6 - 8 minutes. Close the waffle maker.
4. Check after about 5 minutes. Cook until crisp.
5. Take out the chaffle and set aside on a plate. Let it sit for a couple of minutes.
6. Repeat steps 3 – 5 and make the remaining chaffles.

# Easy Chaffle with Keto Sausage Gravy

Makes: 4 servings

## Ingredients:

<u>For chaffle:</u>

- 2 eggs
- 2 teaspoons coconut flour
- ½ teaspoon baking powder
- 1 cup grated mozzarella cheese
- 2 teaspoons water
- 1/8 teaspoon salt

<u>For keto sausage gravy:</u>

- ½ pound breakfast sausage
- 4 tablespoons heavy whipping cream
- ½ teaspoon garlic powder
- ½ teaspoon onion powder (optional)
- 6 tablespoons chicken broth
- 4 teaspoons cream cheese, softened
- Pepper to taste
- Salt to taste

## Directions:

1. For chaffles: Preheat the mini waffle maker.

2. Add eggs into a bowl and whisk well. Add coconut flour, baking powder, mozzarella cheese, water and salt and whisk well. Let the batter sit for 2 minutes.

3. Spoon ¼ of the batter into the waffle maker. Set the timer for about 6 - 8 minutes. Close the waffle maker.

4. Check after about 5 minutes. Cook until crisp.

5. Take out the chaffle and set aside on a plate.

6. Repeat steps 3 – 5 and make the remaining chaffles.

7. To make keto sausage gravy: Place a skillet over medium heat. Add sausage and cook until brown. Use ½ cup of the sausage to make the gravy. Store the remaining in the refrigerator (after cooling) in an airtight container. It can be used in some other recipe.

8. Drain off the fat from the skillet. Add sausage, cream, garlic powder, onion powder if using, chicken broth, cream cheese, salt and pepper and mix well. Place the skillet over medium heat. Stir constantly until it begins to boil.

9. Lower the heat and simmer uncovered until thick.

10. Place the chaffles on individual serving plates. Spread the gravy on the chaffles and serve.

# Japanese Breakfast Chaffle

Makes: 4 chaffles

## Ingredients:

- 1 cup finely shredded mozzarella cheese
- 2 large eggs
- 2 tablespoons Kewpie mayonnaise or regular keto friendly mayonnaise + extra to serve
- 1 slice bacon, chopped
- 2 green onions, sliced

## Directions:

1. Preheat the mini waffle maker.
2. Beat eggs with a fork. Add mayonnaise and stir well.
3. Add half the green onions and bacon into the bowl of egg and stir well.
4. Spoon ¼ of the batter into the waffle maker. Set the timer for 2 to 3 minutes. Sprinkle ¼ cup cheese. Close the waffle maker.
5. Take out the chaffle and set aside on a plate. Let it sit for a couple of minutes.
6. Repeat steps 3 – 4 and make the remaining chaffles.
7. Garnish with remaining green onion and serve some more kewpie mayonnaise.

210

# Cajun and Shrimp Avocado Chaffle

Makes: 2 sandwiches

**Ingredients:**

For chaffle:

- 1 cup shredded part-skim mozzarella cheese
- 2 large eggs
- ½ teaspoon Cajun seasoning

For filling:

- ½ pound raw shrimp, peeled, deveined
- 2 slices bacon, cooked
- 2 tablespoons thinly sliced red onion
- ½ teaspoon Cajun seasoning
- ½ tablespoon bacon grease
- 1 medium avocado, peeled, pitted, sliced
- 4 tablespoons cream cheese, softened
- 1 scallion, minced
- 1 tablespoon bacon bits

**Directions:**

1. Preheat the mini waffle maker.

2. Beat eggs and Cajun seasoning with a fork. Stir in the mozzarella.

3. Spoon ¼ of the batter into the waffle maker. Set the timer for 2 to 3 minutes. Close the waffle maker.

4. Take out the chaffle and set aside on a plate. Let it sit for a couple of minutes.

5. Repeat steps 3 – 4 and make the remaining chaffles.

6. To make filling: Add shrimp, salt, pepper and Cajun seasoning into a bowl. Toss well.

7. Place a skillet over medium heat. Add bacon grease. Add the shrimp mixture and cook until shrimp turns pink. Turn off the heat.

8. To make cream cheese spread: Add cream cheese, scallions and bacon bits into a bowl and whisk well.

9. To assemble: Spread a tablespoon of the cream cheese spread on each of the chaffles. Place 2 chaffles on a serving platter. Divide the filling and place over the chaffles. Cover with the remaining 2 chaffles and serve.

# Keto Sausage Omelet Chaffle

Makes: 2 chaffles

## Ingredients:

- 1 egg
- ½ teaspoon minced onion
- 2 tablespoons finely shredded cheese of your choice
- 2 mini sausages
- ½ teaspoon diced tomatoes
- ½ teaspoon diced green pepper
- Salt to taste
- Pepper to taste

## Directions:

1. Whisk together eggs, salt and pepper in a bowl. Add tomato, onion and bell pepper and stir.
2. Stir in the mozzarella cheese.
3. Spoon ½ the batter into the waffle maker. Set the timer for 2 to 3 minutes. Close the waffle maker.
4. Take out the chaffle and set aside on a plate. Let it sit for a couple of minutes.
5. Repeat steps 3 – 4 and make the remaining chaffles.
6. Place mini sausage on 2 of the chaffles. Cover with the remaining 2 chaffles and serve.

214

# Sausage and Egg Chaffle Sandwich

Makes: 2 sandwiches

**Ingredients:**

<u>For chaffle:</u>

- 2 eggs
- 2 tablespoons almond flour
- 1 cup mozzarella or Monterey Jack cheese
- 4 tablespoons butter

<u>For filling:</u>

- Eggs, cooked as per your preference (fried or omelet or scrambled)
- 2 mini sausage patties
- 2 slices cheese
- 4 tablespoons keto friendly mayonnaise

**Directions:**

1. Preheat the mini waffle maker.
2. Spoon ¼ of the batter into the waffle maker. Set the timer for 3 to 4 minutes. Close the waffle maker.
3. Take out the chaffle and set aside on a plate.
4. Repeat steps 2 – 3 and make the remaining chaffles.

5. Place a skillet over medium heat. Add 2 tablespoons butter. When butter melts, place 2 chaffles and until crisp. Press lightly while cooking. Flip sides and cook the other side until crisp.

6. Remove onto a plate. Let it rest for a couple of minutes before serving.

7. Spread a tablespoon of mayonnaise on each chaffle. Place a sausage patties and a slice of cheese on each. Cover with the remaining chaffles and serve.

# Chapter 5: Keto Pizza Chaffle Recipes

## Keto Pizza Chaffle # 1

Makes: 4 chaffles

**Ingredients:**

- 2 eggs
- ¼ teaspoon Italian seasoning or to taste
- 1 cup shredded mozzarella cheese

To top:

- Pepperoni slices
- Shredded mozzarella cheese
- 2 – 3 tablespoons keto friendly pizza sauce
- 

**Directions:**

1. For chaffles: Preheat the mini waffle maker.
2. Add eggs into a bowl and whisk well. Add Italian seasoning and whisk well.
3. Add mozzarella cheese and whisk well. Let the batter sit for 2 minutes.

4. Spoon ¼ of the batter into the waffle maker. Set the timer for about 6 - 8 minutes. Close the waffle maker.

5. Check after about 5 minutes. Cook until crisp.

6. Take out the chaffle and set aside on a plate.

7. Repeat steps 4 – 6 and make the remaining chaffles.

8. Spread pizza sauce on top of the chaffles. Sprinkle cheese. Place pepperoni slices.

9. Place in the microwave and cook on high for 20 seconds.

# Keto Pizza Chaffle # 2

Makes: 4 chaffles

## Ingredients:

- 2 eggs
- ½ teaspoon dried basil or to taste
- 1 cup shredded mozzarella cheese
- 1 teaspoon baking powder
- ½ teaspoon garlic powder
- 2 tablespoons almond flour

To top:

- 4 tablespoons shredded mozzarella cheese
- 4 tablespoons keto friendly pasta sauce or pizza sauce

## Directions:

1. For chaffles: Preheat the mini waffle maker.
2. Add eggs into a bowl and whisk well. Add dried basil, almond flour, baking powder and garlic powder and whisk well.
3. Add mozzarella cheese and whisk well. Let the batter sit for 2 minutes.

4. Spoon ¼ of the batter into the waffle maker. Set the timer for about 6 - 8 minutes. Close the waffle maker.

5. Check after about 5 minutes. Cook until crisp.

6. Take out the chaffle and set aside on a plate.

7. Repeat steps 4 – 6 and make the remaining chaffles.

8. Spread a tablespoon of pasta sauce on top of each of the chaffles. Sprinkle a tablespoon of cheese on each.

9. Bake in a preheated oven at 375°F for about 5 minutes or until cheese melts and is brown at a few spots.

# Keto Pizza Chaffle # 3

Makes: 4 chaffles

**Ingredients:**

- 2 egg whites
- ½ teaspoon basil seasoning
- 1 cup shredded mozzarella cheese
- ½ teaspoon baking powder
- ¼ teaspoon garlic powder
- 2 teaspoons coconut flour
- 2 teaspoons cream cheese, softened
- ¼ teaspoon Italian seasoning
- Salt to taste

For topping:

- 6 teaspoons keto friendly marinara sauce
- 12 pepperonis, halved
- ½ teaspoon basil seasoning
- 1 cup shredded mozzarella cheese
- 2 tablespoons shredded Parmesan cheese

**Directions:**

1. For chaffles: Preheat the mini waffle maker.

2. Add egg whites, basil seasoning, Italian seasoning, coconut flour, baking powder, cream cheese, mozzarella cheese, salt and garlic powder into a bowl and whisk well. Let the batter sit for 2 minutes.

3. Spoon ¼ of the batter into the waffle maker. Set the timer for about 6 - 8 minutes. Close the waffle maker.

4. Check after about 5 minutes. Cook until crisp.

5. Take out the chaffle and set aside on a plate.

6. Repeat steps 3 – 5 and make the remaining chaffles.

7. Spread 1-½ tablespoons of marinara sauce on top of each of the chaffles. Sprinkle Parmesan cheese and mozzarella cheese on each. Divide the pepperoni halves among the chaffles and place on top.

8. Bake in a preheated oven at 375°F for about 5 minutes or until cheese melts.

9. Set the oven to broil mode and broil for a couple of minutes. Garnish with basil seasoning and serve.

## Keto Pizza Chaffle # 4

Makes: 1 chaffle

**Ingredients:**

- 1 large egg

- ½ teaspoon baking powder
- ¼ teaspoon garlic powder
- ½ teaspoon basil seasoning
- ¼ cup shredded mozzarella cheese
- ¼ cup shredded cheddar cheese
- 2 tablespoons blanched almond flour
- ¼ teaspoon Italian seasoning
- Salt to taste

For topping:

- 4 teaspoons keto friendly marinara sauce
- 4 mini pepperonis
- ¼ cup shredded mozzarella cheese
- 4 tablespoons shredded Parmesan cheese
- ½ teaspoon freshly chopped basil
- 3 cherry tomatoes, halved
- ¼ bell pepper, diced
- 1 mushroom, sliced

**Directions:**

1. For chaffles: Preheat the regular waffle maker.
2. Add egg, Italian seasoning, almond flour, baking powder and garlic powder into a bowl and whisk well.

3. Add mozzarella cheese and cheddar cheese and stir. Let the batter sit for 2 minutes.

4. Spoon the batter into the waffle maker. Set the timer for about 6 - 8 minutes. Close the waffle maker.

5. Flip sides after 6 minutes. Cook until crisp.

6. Take out the chaffle and set aside on a plate.

7. Spread marinara sauce on top of the chaffles. Sprinkle Parmesan cheese and mozzarella cheese on each. Place mini pepperoni slices place on top. Scatter cherry tomatoes, bell pepper and mushrooms on top.

8. Bake in a preheated oven at 375°F for about 5 minutes or until cheese melts.

9. Set the oven to broil mode and broil for a couple of minutes.

# Conclusion

As we come to an end, I would like to thank you for purchasing this book. I hope you find it useful.

Now you can whip up some delicious keto chaffles whenever you want. They're just as good, if not better than your traditional waffles, but they'll help you stick to a healthy ketogenic diet. So stop waiting and start trying out the yummy recipes in the book. You'll love these breakfast recipes, and so will anyone you make them for.

So what are you waiting for? Let us get started!

www.ingramcontent.com/pod-product-compliance
Lightning Source LLC
Chambersburg PA
CBHW051719020426
42333CB00014B/1057